Losing Me, While Losing You

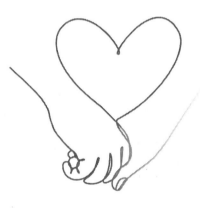

Losing Me, While Losing You

Caregivers Share Their Experiences of Supporting Friends and Family with Dementia

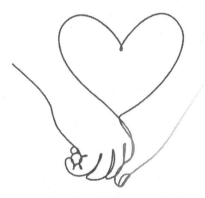

Jeanette A Auger,
Diane Tedford-Litle and
Brenda Wallace-Allen

Fernwood Publishing
Halifax & Winnipeg

Editing: Lisa Frenette
Text design: Brenda Conroy
Cover design: John van der Woude
Printed and bound in Canada

Published by Fernwood Publishing
32 Oceanvista Lane, Black Point, Nova Scotia, B0J 1B0
and 748 Broadway Avenue, Winnipeg, Manitoba, R3G 0X3
www.fernwoodpublishing.ca

Fernwood Publishing Company Limited gratefully acknowledges the financial support of the Government of Canada, the Canada Council for the Arts, the Manitoba Department of Culture, Heritage and Tourism under the Manitoba Publishers Marketing Assistance Program and the Province of Manitoba, through the Book Publishing Tax Credit, for our publishing program. We are pleased to work in partnership with the Province of Nova Scotia to develop and promote our creative industries for the benefit of all Nova Scotians.

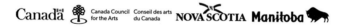

Library and Archives Canada Cataloguing in Publication

Title: Losing me, while losing you: caregivers share their experiences of supporting friends and family with dementia / by Jeanette A. Auger, Diane Tedford-Litle and Brenda Wallace-Allen; foreword by Janice Keefe.
Names: Auger, Jeanette A., 1945- author. | Tedford-Litle, Diane, author. | Wallace-Allen, Brenda, author. | Keefe, Janice, 1963- writer of foreword.
Description: Includes bibliographical references.
Identifiers: Canadiana (print) 20210259558 | Canadiana (ebook) 20210259701 | ISBN 9781773634845 (softcover) | ISBN 9781773635019 (EPUB) | ISBN 9781773635026 (PDF)
Subjects: LCSH: Dementia—Patients—Care. | LCSH: Dementia—Patients—Family relationships. | LCSH: Caregivers.
Classification: LCC RC521 .A94 2021 | DDC 362.1968/31—dc23

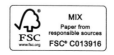

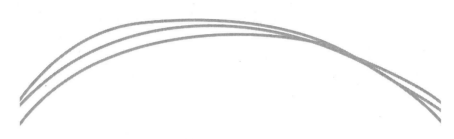

Contents

Acknowledgements

We sincerely thank the caregivers who so openly shared their experiences with us, especially in the difficult time of a pandemic, and who did so because they wanted their experiences to be shared with others who may have similar experiences now and in the future.

From Fernwood, we thank Errol Sharpe for his continued support and encouragement of our endeavours. As well, we appreciate Beverley Rach, who once again guided us through the publishing process. Our thanks go to Lisa Frenette, who was our copy editor, Debbie Mathers and to Brenda Conroy for her involvement and expertise, which always make our work so much better.

We thank our friend and computer guru Terry Aulenbach for ensuring that all the correct publishing guidelines were met and adhered to and for doing so with patience.

We thank each other for our support and understanding as we each experienced health care challenges while going through the research and writing process, but we were determined to share the experiences of the caregivers for whom we have so much respect and admiration.

Kirstie Creighton, manager for Program Development at the Alzheimer Society of Nova Scotia, was very helpful in providing resources, and we thank her for her considerate attention to our requests. Dr. Janice Keefe, chair of the Nova Scotia Centre on Aging at Mount Saint Vincent University and chair of the provincial expert panel on long-term care in Nova Scotia, kindly agreed to write the foreword to this book, and we are deeply gateteful that this very busy, proficient and prolific woman took time to do this.

Foreword

Alzheimer's disease and other related dementias have rightly gained importance in the academic milieu as well as our day-to-day society. In Nova Scotia alone, it is estimated that nineteen thousand people develop dementia every year. *Losing Me While Losing You* is an insightful entry into the lives of the people who care for persons with dementia. Caregivers have often been called the backbone of our health care system, supporting those who need assistance.

In Canada, 80 percent of the support provided to older people in need of assistance comes from family and friends. The care provided to persons living with dementia by their family and friends enables them to live far longer in the community than would be possible. Even when care needs become so great that nursing home admission is needed, family continue to provide essential emotional and physical support and contribute to their quality of life. The knowledge gained through interviewing caregivers is critical to help improve support for both the caregivers and the persons with a dementia diagnosis.

The organization of this book follows the stages of the journey as seen through the eyes of the caregivers: Noticin g, Responding, Assistance and Support, and Observations and Recommendations. Chapter 6 is a compendium of resources and supports available to caregivers. There are many strengths to the content — one is diversity of the caregivers interviewed. They represent different ethnic and cultural experiences, and they have a variety of living arrangements, geographies, education and relationships with the person they are caring for — be they wives and husbands, mothers and fathers, from large families or small.

Not so long ago, it was taboo to speak about our experiences of dementia — the "noticing stage" that the authors bring to life through the words of the caregivers help us to identify the multiple ways in which the disease is first manifest. In the recent past we would have been in denial of the disease, afraid that by speaking about it we will it to happen or somehow it is the fault of the person with dementia. Indeed, some groups may still be in denial because of fear, because they feel that nothing can be done to turn the tide of dementia progression. Nothing could be further from the truth. Some types of dementia can be stabilized through medication. For others, the knowledge of cognitive impairment provides an opportunity for family and the person with the diagnosis to discuss future plans and preferences. Rather than hide behind closed doors, the thirty-five caregivers in this book offer insights into the process of noticing, how they responded and their encounters, good and bad, of seeking assistance and support.

The wealth of information on support and resources throughout the book will be beneficial to anyone who is currently a caregiver or is studying how to support people with dementia and their caregivers. Caregivers provide insightful recommendations on lessons learned, coping strategies and what government can do to best support caregivers. The positive personal growth caregivers experienced through their journeys is another valuable lesson from the book — one that is often overlooked in research literature.

From the personal to the societal response, the authors' descriptions of the caregivers' experiences reveal a patchwork of programs and services in Nova Scotia. This is in contrast to the long history of national dementia strategies across the globe and across the provinces within Canada. The chapter on resources is comprehensive in its examination of leading-edge initiatives such as dementia villages, dementia-friendly communities, memory care facilities, geriatric clinics and a host of other initiatives. It also tackles the under-recognized topics of the impact of race and ethnicity on dementia care. Understanding the intent and scope of these resources is essential for anyone working in this field.

Losing Me, While Losing You brings to life essential knowledge to support family and friend caregivers in caring for persons with a dementia diagnosis. I am very grateful to the thirty-five caregivers who shared their stories with us and the insights they have for others who find themselves on this dementia journey. Finally, thank you to the authors who chose a narrative approach to write these reflections and organized the vast material in an accessible way for all to read.

— Janice M. Keefe, PhD, professor and chair, Department of Family Studies and Gerontology, Lena Isabel Jodrey Chair in Gerontology, director, Nova Scotia Centre on Aging, Mount Saint Vincent University, April 2021

Preface

As older women moving about in our communities of family, friends, acquaintances and others, we became increasingly concerned about the numbers of persons we knew or heard about who had been diagnosed with dementia, including Alzheimer's disease. We also heard many stories about the challenging experiences of caregivers of persons living with dementia, usually within their own homes. As we are engaged advocates for ourselves and other older persons and because we have taught, researched, published and engaged in community development activities with and for older persons and their important ones in a variety of settings, we were interested in hearing more about how such work impacts the caregiver's sense of self in relation to the person with dementia. For example, in October of 2019, Jeanette had a conversation with a friend about her experience of caring for her husband with dementia. The friend said,

> *We have been married for forty-two years. I was his wife, his lover and best friend, mother of his children and confidant. I was also his memory keeper. Now he doesn't know who I am and it is like I have been erased from his life, and mine. So, I don't know who I am anymore either.*

Another friend, who is caring for his wife who has been diagnosed with Alzheimer's disease, made the following remarks:

> *She has really bad memory lapses now, so sometimes she calls me Bob, who was her younger brother. He has been dead for years. Some days I am not sure who I am. I am so tired, so pretending to be Bob is easier to deal with rather than reminding her that it's me, her husband of all these years.*

Diane has a friend whose mother died from sudden-onset Alzheimer's disease twenty years ago. She said that the memories of this loss are as traumatic today as they were at the time:

> *Amid much criticism I had to put my mother in long-term care on doctor's orders. My severe shock came not long after when I arrived at the nursing home and my mother greeted me with "and who are you?" I was an only child and I couldn't believe what was happening. I was in total shock and started to shake all over. A nurse saw my reaction and led me out to the nursing station for comfort. The shock was so great. The woman who had birthed me, loved me, nurtured me had no idea who I was? At that time there was very little help for family members or caregivers to deal with this type of shock and bewilderment. These feelings are just as clear to me today as they were then. I have not recovered from this pain.*

In a 2019 Government of Canada report on dementia, data showed that more than 419,000 Canadians (65 years and older) were living with diagnosed dementia, almost two-thirds of whom were women. As this number does not include those under age 65 who may have a young-onset diagnosis nor those who have not been diagnosed, the true picture of dementia in Canada is no doubt somewhat larger (Government of Canada 2019).

Little did we realize when we began this journey of interviewing care-givers of persons with dementia, that we would do some of this work during a pandemic, when gaining access to potential interviewees would be challenging, especially when they lived in the homes of the persons who were diagnosed, so that entering the home to conduct an interview was not always possible. As a result, some of our interviews were conducted over the telephone and others via email responses to the questions we sent to informants. On other occasions, we conducted interviews outside resi-dences where physical distance could be maintained; in other instances, family members conducted the interviews and then sent them to us.

The COVID-19 pandemic also introduced another component to the lives of caregivers and those they cared for as many experienced isolation, loneliness, anxiety and fear of rejection from neighbours and friends due to the stigma associated with dementia. In some cases, paid caregivers were not comfortable entering homes to provide care and support for fear of contracting the virus, which made caregiving by loved ones even more challenging. Further compounding the need for respite from the twenty-four hours a day, seven days a week care that important ones provide, adult day programs, which offer respite relief for caregivers, were closed due to the pandemic, as were other long-term care facilities which have day programs. Some of the people we interviewed told us that they used to take their loved ones for regular doctor's visits for updates on their conditions, so, as one said, "At least we got to go for a drive for a reason and it was an opportunity to get out of the house." Due to COVID-19, doctor's visits were conducted over the telephone, once again isolating both patients and their caregivers from face-to-face social interaction.

Many with dementia diagnoses who lived in long-term care facilities were not allowed to have visitors, and if and when they were, they could only have a thirty-minute visit once a week by appointment only, and they were not allowed physical contact with their loved ones. For families with many relatives, especially in the case of parents with many children, partners and siblings had to decide when and who would visit, meaning that some did not see their loved ones for many weeks. If family members had others living in their homes who worked outside of the province and they had to self-quarantine for fourteen days when returning home, the entire family could not visit a long-term care home. Residents of such facilities with dementia diagnoses often told their loved ones that they felt rejected and orphaned by their families because they did not understand about the pandemic. In some cases, family members purchased cell phones and laptop computers so that their loved ones could see and talk to them virtually, but many times the person with dementia was unable to comprehend how to use the technology and staff were not always available to assist them with it. One particular story touched us deeply when a man, with six siblings and a 95-year-old mother who was blind, deaf and lived in a nursing home, decided on a creative solution to allow his mother to know which of her children was visiting. While living in her own home prior to her deteriorating health, every Christmas and birthday his mother knitted hats, toques and scarves for each of her children as gifts. He had an old sweater his mother had made for him some years ago, and he placed it in a bag and asked the attendant at the nursing home on his next visit if she would give his mother the sweater, which she agreed to do. When his mother placed the sweater to her face and smelled it, she seemed to know which son was visiting and she broke into tears, as did he and the care worker. We saw this as a sign of resilience and creativity in challenging times.

In spite of our challenges, we continued undaunted with our research and the result is a group of narrative accounts on the experiences of some caregivers of persons diagnosed with dementia, including Alzheimer's disease, in various parts of Nova Scotia. We are grateful to all of them for sharing their difficult and sometimes rewarding experiences with us.

As well as the interviews with caregivers, we conducted a literature search of the material available on this topic, and we also reviewed the demographic and statistical material. Jeanette was asked to discuss this research to a group of university students enrolled in a course on death and dying. In November of 2019, the students were sent background material on the topic and asked to complete a set of questions about dementia. They returned the responses to Jeanette prior to her online discussion with them, and in some cases we have included their responses in the book.

Introduction

To help provide some context for our research on the topic of dementia in Canada we thought it useful to provide some historical and demographic details.

Historical Background of the Terms

The term dementia comes from its Latin roots *demens*, which means out of one's mind. Although this term has been used since the thirteenth century it was not until the eighteenth century that medical practioners in European countries used it to diagnose patients. In the nineteenth century "senile dementia" was originally seen as a separate disease from Alzheimer's but as medical knowledge increased and expanded it became recognized as one of many neuro cognitive disorders (Assal 2019: 118–126).

Alois Alzheimer was a German psychiatrist and neuropathologist who in 1906, noticed changes in the brain tissue of a woman who had died of an unusual mental illness. Her symptoms included memory loss, language problems and unpredictable behaviour. At that time Alzheimer diagnosed his patient as having presenile dementia. Later his colleague Emil Kraepelin would define this condition as Alzheimer's disease (Alzheimer's Disease International n.d.a). Alzheimer's disease is the most common condition resulting in dementia. In 2013 the Diagnostic and Statistical Manual of Mental Disorders (DSM-5) noted that their preferred term for this disorder was "major neurocognitive disorder" in an attempt to help reduce the stigma associated with both the word dementia and the conditions that it refers to. This term has not yet gained popularity even among organizations serving individuals with this diagnosis (Warchol n.d.).

According to the Public Health Agency of Canada,

Dementia is a fatal, progressive and degenerative disease that destroys brain cells. It is caused by neurodegenerative and vascular diseases or injuries. It is characterized by a decline in cognitive abilities and can impact mood and behaviour. The cognitive abilities that can be impacted include:

memory
awareness of person, place and time
language
basic math skills
judgement
planning. (Government of Canada 2019)

Demographics

In 2015, the Nova Scotia Department of Health and Wellness reported: "Today, more than 17,000 Nova Scotians are living with dementia. In the coming years, we expect that number to double as our population continues to age. While the numbers are significant, the impact on the individuals affected and their families can be devastating" (Nova Scotia Department of Health and Wellness 2015: 1).

Alzheimer's Disease International, located in the United Kingdom, notes that more than 50 million people worldwide have been diagnosed with Alzheimer's disease. It is believed that one in four people with the disease have not been diagnosed <Alzheimer's Disease International. n.d.a>.

By 2030 the Alzheimer Society of Canada estimates that the number of Canadians living with dementia will be 912,000. Every year 25,000 more Canadians are diagnosed with dementia. This organization estimates the annual costs of care for persons with dementia is over $12 billion.

Indigenous and Black Canadians, including those living in Nova Scotia are three times more likely to be diagnosed with dementia. For more information on this topic see the report *Alzheimer's Disease and Related Dementias in Indigenous Populations in Canada: Prevalence and Risk Factors,* produced and written by Julia Petrasek MacDonald, Valerie Ward and Regine Halseth, for the National Collaborating Council on Indigenous Health in January 2018, and also the website of the Alzheimer Society of Canada (alzheimer.ca).

Of those diagnosed with dementia, including Alzheimer's disease, 65 percent are women; women make up two-thirds of the caregivers for persons with dementia, and approximately 34 percent of them are aged

65 or older. One in five Canadians have experience in caring for someone living with dementia.

Although the literature on gender differences in Alzheimer's disease diagnoses is scant, there is reasearch to support that factors such as depression, life-long exercise, age and sleep can have an impact on the development of dementia.

There is general agreement among authors that twice as many women as men in North American and European cultures live with depression and that depression can be a precursor to dementia. This is not to say that men do not experience depression, but that women are more likely to seek medical assistance when they do. Another reason posited for the differences is that women, especially in later life, do not exercise as much as men in formal settings such a gyms, hockey stadiums, soccer fields and other community-based sports venues. Because age is also a factor involved in diagnoses of dementia, the fact that women live longer than men is another potential reason why more women than men are diagnosed.

Types of Dementia

There are over two hundred sub types of dementia, according to Dementia UK (n.d.). However, the most commonly diagnosed six are the following:

1. Alzheimer's disease is the most common form of dementia. It is a chronic neurodegenerative disease that destroys brain cells, causing thinking ability and memory to deteriorate over time. Alzheimer's disease is a not a normal part of aging and is irreversible.
2. Vascular dementia is the second most common form. It occurs when the brain's blood supply is blocked or damaged, causing brain cells to be deprived of oxygen and die.
3. Lewy body dementia is caused by abnormal "Lewy bodies," which are deposits of protein called alpha-synuclein inside of the brain's nerve cells. This type of dementia shares many similarities to Parkinson's disease.
4. Frontotemporal dementia (also known as Pick's disease) is an umbrella term for a group of rare disorders that primarily affect the areas of the brain associated with personality and behaviour.
5. Young-onset dementia is the term used to describe people under the age of 65 who are diagnosed with this disease. It can also be called early-onset dementia.

6. Mixed dementia is the term used when people have more than one type of dementia.

Limbic-predominant age-related TDP-43 (LATE-NC) is the most recently identified form of dementia, noted for its close similarity to Alzheimer's disease. When TDP-43 accumulates in an area located in the mid-brain known as the limbic system, it affects learning, memory and emotion, resembling symptoms of Alzheimer's disease, the most common form of dementia. This suggests that people may exhibit symptoms mirroring those of Alzheimer's but may not involve the same changes to the brain caused by the disease. Currently, LATE-NC is not diagnosable with standard tests. Because people are typically diagnosed with certain types of dementia based on the symptoms they experience, LATE-NC will not be easily distinguished from Alzheimer's due to overlapping symptoms. Further research is required to improve diagnosis in identifying the different diseases that can lead to dementia, including LATE-NC. Investigators are currently trying to understand how to identify and diagnose LATE-NC clinically. The discovery of LATE-NC speaks to the growing umbrella of different dementias and the complexity of these diseases (Alzheimer Society of Canada 2019b).

The Research

In order to collect the experiences of caregivers of persons with dementia we used a snowball sampling technique. We each knew people who acted in these roles and they knew others in similar situations, either through being involved in research initiatives attempting to find cures for dementia, such as the True North Medical Research Clinics, through adult day programs, where they received respite care, or through word of mouth when discussing their situation with others who shared their experiences. We also posted information about the research on social media and contacted Alzheimer and dementia support group leaders, some of whom passed on the information to groups that were meeting online during the pandemic. As well, some of the students with whom Jeanette interacted said that they had experiences with loved ones with Alzheimer's and agreed to participate in the research by completing questionnaires online.

The Questionnaire

We asked a total of twenty-two questions (See Appendix A). The first set of questions asked for basic information such as the name, sex, age and race of the interviewee and the person they were caring for as well as their relationship status, such as parent, partner, child, friend and so on. We wanted to know when they first noticed changes in the behaviours of the person they were caring for and what they did about it; when the person was first diagnosed and their age at the time; what roles the person and the interviewee played in their relationship with each other; if the roles for each changed during the progression of the disease and if so in what ways; if any respite care was provided to the caregiver and if so, who provided the care; if the caregiver experienced stress or burnout or felt overworked as they pursued their caregiving responsibilities; how the role changes have impacted their lives; whether or not their incomes were affected; and how the community, other family members and friends have responded to the person's dementia. We asked if the caregivers learned anything about themselves as a result of their experiences caring for an important one, as well as whether they perceived benefits due to this work. We asked if their faith contributed to their experiences, what coping strategies they used to assist them in these challenging roles and how the experience has affected how they feel about themselves. Finally, we asked if the caregivers had any recommendations they could provide to others in similar situations and whether or not there were other issues we had not dealt with that they would like to expand upon or share.

The interviews lasted between one to two or more hours. Most were held in caregivers homes, but due to the COVID-19 pandemic we also conducted interviews in the grounds of long-term care facilities, over the telephone, through emailed questionnaires and via friends who were sent the interview questions and then conducted the interviews, transcribed them and returned them to us. In some cases, caregivers showed us photographs of their weddings, grandchildren, awards the person with dementia had received and other evidence of their lives together. Our youngest interviewee showed us woodworking projects he and his grandfather had worked on when he was well.

In order to ensure confidentiality, we have not used the real names of interviewees, unless they specifically said we could, which happened in a few cases. Instead we asked them to choose a pseudonym, and most did, including some who made comments like "I have never liked my name and am happy to choose another," or "I have always liked the name X and wanted to call my daughter that, but my husband wanted her to have his mother's name."

The interviews were at times deeply emotional for the caregivers as well as us and tears were often shed when remembering better times. COVID-19 further complicated the situation as it was not clear when family could visit again, when a nursing home bed might become available as the person with dementia's condition deteriorated and when respite or home care would become more readily available.

We were very moved and thankful that in these times of the pandemic people were willing to share their experiences with us — in some cases the person with dementia would be present during the interviews so there were stoppages in the conversations as they needed to be attended to. In spite of their work as caregivers, we were often provided with cups of tea, baked goods and even, on a few occasions, lunch. Due to the pandemic and the feelings of loneliness and isolation experienced by some of the caregivers, some said our presence provided a friendly and caring visit and change of pace for them.

The Interviewees

Age Range of Participants

In total we conducted full interviews with thirty-five people; the majority were female, and five were male. The ages of caregivers ranged from 11 (the youngest) to an 89-year-old (the oldest). The majority were in their sixties, seventies and eighties, and some interviewees did not supply their age as they did not consider it significant to the questions asked.

Race and Ethnicity of Participants

The majority of our interviews were conducted with persons who self-identified as Caucasian. We also conducted one interview with a Chinese couple, four with people who identified as African Nova Scotian, three with people who identified as Indigenous and one as East Indian. In order to further discuss the situation regarding Indigenous and African Nova Scotians we relied on a literature search and recent material (2020) compiled by the Alzheimer Society of Nova Scotia and the National Collaborating Centre for Aboriginal Health in Prince George, British Columbia. Some of this material is discussed later in the book.

Diagnoses

The majority of people we interviewed were caring for persons who had been diagnosed with Alzheimer's disease. Others were diagnosed with unspecified dementia, vascular dementia, frontal lobe dementia, Parkinson's disease dementia and dementia with Lewy bodies. In addition, one caregiver shared that her mother's dementia was the result of medication, and in another case the dementia was brought on by radiation of the brain.

Who Was Being Cared For

The majority provided care for their mothers. Others provided care for their husbands, wives, fathers, mothers-in-law and grandfathers. One provided care for a father-in-law, one for herself, another for a grandmother and another for a friend.

Location of Care

The majority ended their caregiving journey providing care in a long-term care facility, such as a nursing home. Fourteen were providing care in their own homes or the home of the individual living with dementia, and two stories involved admission into hospitals where the individuals awaited transfers to long-term care homes when beds became available.

The Geographic Locations of Interviewees

The interviews were conducted in a variety of settings across the province of Nova Scotia with the majority being in the HRM (Halifax Regional Municipality) and Kings County. Interviews were also conducted in Cape Breton, Mahone Bay, Preston and Shelburne, and others identified as living in "rural areas." Some interviewees preferred not to provide their location to protect their anonymity.

Present Caregiving Situation or Remembering Ones From the Past

The majority of interviewees were providing care to their important ones at the time of the interviews and had been doing so from one to five years or more. In some cases, the person with dementia had died and the person interviewed was recalling their experiences and reflections since the death of their loved one from one to eighteen years ago, with the majority in the past five years.

The Themes

In order to present the narrative accounts of providing care to an important one living with dementia, we broke the interviews down into four distinct themes. The first we call "Noticing," which addresses the warning signs caregivers observed when their loved ones started to experience memory loss, confusion, agitation or other symptoms associated with various forms of dementia. In this theme caregivers share their experiences of being in denial, resisting the new roles imposed on them by the disease and their attempts to get a proper diagnosis.

The second theme we identified as "Responding." In this chapter of the book the caregivers share the ways in which they attempted to access resources; the impacts on their own health and wellness; the challenges they faced in regard to loneliness, fear, exhaustion and assuming new roles; and how these changes impacted their images of self.

In the third theme, "Assistance and Support," the caregivers focus on the support they did, or did not receive from others, including professionals, and the lessons they learned as they conducted their work. They also talk about what they would have done differently had circumstances allowed and the ways in which the health care system needs to change to support caregivers more adequately.

The fourth theme focuses on "Observations and Recommendations" and is where the caregivers share with us which strategies they found helpful in the care they provided, as well as the recommendations they would make to government and others in similar situations.

In Chapter 6 we examine some of the gaps that have existed in dementia care locally, in the Candian context and internationally, and we discuss ways in which these gaps are being addressed. We conclude the book with a brief chapter titled "Losing Me."

Introducing the Caregivers

Rather than repeat the information about each caregiver as we discuss their experiences, we thought it best to introduce you to them at the start of their narratives. In each case we give you the name of the caregiver, age (where provided), name of the person being cared for and their relationship to the caregiver. We also provide the location of where they were living when the interview was conducted. Rather than provide specific geographic locations we identify them more generally to provide confidentiality — for example the greater Halifax Regional Municipality, or a small town in Kings County, or Cape Breton, unless the interviewee specifically asked for their location to be made known.

In addition to in-depth interviews with the thirty-five caregivers, we also gathered information from a class of students at a Halifax university and three Indigenous women who provide care professionally as well as providing support to family members with dementia.

The Text Within

Because the caregivers we interviewed were so willing to share their experiences with us, we felt it appropriate that we also share our personal stories of family and friends who have experienced and do experience dementia.

Diane's Story

As I took part in interviews with folks taking care of loved ones with dementia I had time to reflect on my experience with family members who lived with dementia in their later years.

My paternal grandmother, a widow and former missionary in India, developed dementia later in her life. She took to singing off key while playing a piano and later on had hallucinations. My uncle and his wife arranged for my grandmother to be admitted to a Roman Catholic long-term care facility and then left to retire to British Columbia. My mother and father had been in a horrific accident and had left the city to live in rural Nova Scotia. At the time of Grammy's developing dementia I was left as the only living relative in the city. I was newly married and expecting our first child. For several years I only got to visit my grandmother several times a year. I had no idea what was really going on. It was several years later on a visit that I discovered that my grandmother was given antibiotics for several cases of pneumonia. By this time she was a living "corpse" and not able to function on her own in any way. I was horrified that she was being kept alive. I objected to the use of antibiotics and finally Grammy died peacefully.

Then my uncle developed dementia, having served in World War II. I remember on my last visit to him in BC, we went for a walk and he stated to me, "It is so disturbing to realize my brother's (my father's) body is totally wearing out but his mind is still intact while my body is strong and my mind is going."

I remember his wife leaving notes around the house and my uncle buying bricks of ice cream. The freezer was full of ice cream (his love on returning from the war).

At the time of our last visit I was a volunteer palliative care worker in the Valley. I was particularly upset as Joy (his wife) continued to insist my uncle stay at home. I remember her telling me at times she would curl up in the middle of the floor to avoid my uncle's rage. When he was finally admitted to long-term care she still insisted he be force-fed! I was mortified! Finally members of the palliative care team talked to her and explained what would be most beneficial for her loved one. My uncle finally died in peace several months later.

I am now 82 and had major surgery last August from which I am recovering. When I forgot a name at first I would worry that I was developing dementia, but now I have come to realize stress doesn't help. I simply laugh now and say to myself, "Oh well, I will remember a little later" and I usually do! I am doing okay living alone through this COVID-19 pandemic!

Jeanette's Story

I have been fortunate to not have anyone in my immediate family be diagnosed with dementia, to my knowledge. However, I have had very good friends and neighbours diagnosed with dementia over the years. In fact, it was the experience of one such friend which piqued my interest and concern about the experience of being the caregiver for a loved one with dementia. I watched this couple first deal with the husband's diagnosis after he had several memory tests that showed he had a slight decline in memory, to a year later him being diagnosed with dementia and then experiencing a fast decline as the disease progressed. I watched his wife of forty-two years struggle with trying to find appropriate care for her husband, especially respite, which was booked but then cancelled after a three-month wait. In the end, their son who lives in Scotland convinced them to leave Nova Scotia and go and live there so that they could receive better care. They did do this, in spite of living in this province for twenty-five years after moving here from the UK.

After their arrival in a small town in Scotland, the husband became agitated and angry and was using aggressive behaviour towards his wife. As a result, first he was placed in a hospital and then in a private nursing home; he has been institutionalized. Due to the pandemic and her own poor health, which she attributes to the stress of caring for her husband, his wife was unable to visit him for three months. She is now able to do so for half an hour a week, all without being able to physically touch him with a hug or a kiss. She says his condition has deteriorated since he was first admitted into the care facility, to the point that he doesn't always recognize her, their son and his wife, or his three-year-old granddaughter.

Many years ago, a dear friend was diagnosed with young-onset Alzheimer's at 50 years of age. I watched as her partner of thirty years cared for her and tried to keep their life as "normal" as possible in spite of the many challenges involved in being a main caregiver. Two years after her diagnosis she was admitted into a care facility, where she died two months later.

I have several neighbours who have had partners diagnosed with dementia. Three have died — one very recently. I have observed and been party to the challenges all of these people have bravely taken on to ensure that their important ones receive the best care available to them, all while losing sight of the need to care for their own health in the process. In most cases the caregivers ended up needing care. As well, I have learned from them all that when a loved one has dementia and becomes invisible to themselves, and sometimes others, that the caregivers struggle with their own identity and self-esteem.

Recently a friend, whose husband died in a nursing home from Alzheimer's disease, said of her sense of self, "It's as if I look into a mirror which has broken and see shattered bits of myself all over the place since he has been gone. It used to be when I looked I saw a wife, mother, grandmother, dresser (I always dressed him as he had no sense of style otherwise), cook and cleaner. I was his constant companion and I would say his oldest and best friend. Now I look in the mirror and see so much is gone. So after losing him, I only hope I can find me again." These experiences are why I wanted to co-write this book.

Brenda's Story

I have worked with aging people and taught gerontology courses throughout my career. When I was younger the challenges presented by aging were opportunities to explore new approaches and new ways of doing things. I liked teaming with older people and learning from them as we conducted research and developed new programs. I had older people among my close circle of friends, and I admired their keen minds, fearless advocacy efforts and commitment to make changes in their lives and their communities when needed.

I met my "Waterloo" when working (and living) with older people involved the challenge of dementia in my own family. Both my father-in-law and father developed dementia. My father-in-law had Parkinson's disease, and in addition to changes in his cognitive functioning he lost his wonderfully expressive face which was replaced by a "Parkinsonian mask."

My father had dementia which was originally diagnosed as Alzheimer's disease but was likely vascular dementia. He died two years ago.

As I was growing up my father had a brilliant mind and was an eloquent speaker. His storytelling was always relatable and didactic. My mother was the first to notice that something was not right and that his forgetfulness might be more than what would be typical for his age. My father described his forgetfulness as "bobbing for apples" — you know they (the words) are in there and if you keep trying you will eventually bite into the right word and emerge triumphant.

As the dementia progressed his communication became more like attempting to put together a jigsaw puzzle. He appeared to see the total picture, but he only communicated with us in pieces and most often some of the key pieces were missing.

What I found more frustrating than my father's reduced level of communication was the resignation that accompanied the dementia. He was still interested in the things happening around him, but he was not interested in, nor capable of, initiating things or making them happen. This had been the part of my father that I had always admired. He would come up with unique, cutting edge ideas and he would then do everything to move those ideas forward.

As I adjusted to my father's changing capacities it reminded me of a fabulous sandcastle as the tide comes in. With each wave more and more of the castle is worn away until you are left simply remembering what the castle looked like in its glory.

So, I am sharing the concerns raised by watching the slow but progressive downward journey of these two important men in my life. What can we do to prevent dementia? What can be done to reduce the stigma of dementia? What can we do to ensure that caregivers supporting people with dementia are getting the support they need? What changes need to be made to maintain the personhood of those living with dementia in long-term care? How can we best accommodate the end-of-life wishes of persons with dementia?

My starting point is to collect the perspectives, ideas and insights of the persons for whom adjusting to the demands of dementia has also been their lived experience.

Noticing

In the first set of questions we asked the caregivers, we asked them when they first noticed changes in the behaviour of the important one for whom they were caring. Part of that discussion included them recounting what they defined as "warning signs" that gave them some indication that the behaviours being exhibited were more than just, as many noted, "senior moments" or "normal forgetfulness in older people." As a result of witnessing these changes many said that they, and the person they were caring for, were in "denial" that the symptoms could be related to dementia. Once the disease was diagnosed they spoke about the difficulties in receiving a diagnosis for their loved one, and then how they, and the person diagnosed, resisted the new roles which each had to perform in the relationship.

In the online class in which Jeanette discussed this topic with a group of students at a Halifax university, one student remarked:

When younger people forget something we say it's because we had a bad night or were stressed, but when older people forget something we say that they are having a senior moment and it causes us to be in denial about what else might be going on. Before my Gran was diagnosed with dementia the family was in denial and we would joke that Gran was just having another senior moment. When she was diagnosed we all felt so guilty.

Another, who works at a long-term care facility outside of HRM, said,

There is this myth out there that forgetting is a normal part of aging. My grandfather who is in his eighties belongs to a bridge club where most of the players are in their seventies and eighties and you need great memory powers to play bridge. It's another stereotype about old people that we need to get rid of, especially if we want to be able to tell the difference between mild memory losses and dementia.

Here are the caregiver narratives:

Amber

Amber reluctantly agreed to be interviewed at the suggestion of a friend because she didn't "want to dredge up all that pain again," but she also felt it important that people know "how dreadful this disease is and how much people suffer when someone you love has it." Amber is a 57-year-old African Nova Scotian who lives in a small, mainly Black community in Kings County. Amber's mother Joeleen died at their home of "dementia-related causes" two years ago. Joeleen was 73 years of age at the time of her death. Amber was her primary caregiver with support from the VON.

Amber is an only child. As she explained, "Mom got pregnant with me when she was really young; it was her first time having sex and bingo, didn't she end up with me. The guy who got her pregnant just refused to have anything to do with her when she told him." Because of her pregnancy, Joeleen did not complete high school but was able to get a job in a small grocery store near her community. Because the community where she grew up was somewhat closed and her father refused to acknowledge her, Amber and her mother had limited support outside of her maternal grandmother, with whom they lived.

When Amber started to go to school Joeleen attended community college and completed grade 12. After graduating from high school Joeleen got a job in a hardware store in a nearby town and was later promoted as the "housewares manager at the store."

When her grandmother died, that left only Amber and her mother. "Besides being my mom," Amber observed, "she was my best friend. We went to the movies together, shopping, cooking. We went for drives and a few times went on trips together. Mom had a brother who had moved to Toronto and one time we drove there to see him."

Joeleen first started to display symptoms of dementia in her mid-sixties when she started to forget words and the names of people and places. Joeleen herself noticed this at work when she was trying to add items to the list of things which needed to be replenished and would have to ask others in the store what things were called. Amber said this really upset her because her mother was so happy in her work and did not want to lose her job. After a year or two of constantly forgetting people, places and names Amber convinced her mother to see her GP.

The GP sent her for memory tests and as a result she was diagnosed with "mild symptoms of dementia." The GP wasn't sure if things would get worse. He didn't give her any sort of medication and said she should just keep track of how things went along and whether she started to forget more things.

Over the next two years Joeleen

> *just started to get confused and really forgetful. The manager at the store had to talk to her about her forgetting things and talked her into going back to the doctor. In the beginning she was so scared to do that but when things got really bad and she never knew what day it was and whether she was supposed to go to work or not that day, she agreed to see him again. This time he did put her on some pills — Aricept was the name of them. It was supposed to manage the chemicals in the brain, something like that. In the beginning it seemed to work, but later it didn't. Mom was 69 when she was first diagnosed, and she died four years later. Mom always took care of me and then when she got sick, I took care of her and I became the mom.*

Annabelle

Annabelle's mother, Betsey, was "raised" in the residential school in Shubenacadie. When she returned to the reserve she felt that she did not fit in. She was later diagnosed with PTSD and "borderline personality disorder." She started to show signs of dementia very early on but "we were in denial because she was so young." Annabelle speculates that her mother's dementia "may have progressed faster because of these underlying concerns."

Anne

Anne is a former social worker, the single mom of two adult children and recently retired from teaching. Her father, Malcolm (Mac), was diagnosed with Alzheimer's disease and for years she arranged for his care. Eventually he went into a long-term care facility, where he died some years later.

When her father first started to show signs of dementia, Anne was living in British Columbia and was not around her father enough to notice the subtle changes. In pictures that her mother sent, Anne started to notice a change in her father's face — he seemed a bit vacant.

Anne moved back to Nova Scotia just after her dad had a heart attack. At this point she found his responses to questions vague, but she thought that this was possibly caused by the changes in his health and medication. Anne located to a small community about an hour's drive from her parents.

It was not until a bit later that she observed the first really significant change in her father's behaviour. Her parents came to see her in a new home. They both came in and put their coats in the closet and within minutes her father put his jacket on again to leave. Following that she started to notice her mother compensating for changes in her father. When he was not as engaged with activities or conversations Anne's mother, Shirley, became more engaged and in fact spoke for Malcolm. She noticed that her mother had become a terrible backseat driver and Anne spoke to her about how bossy she had become. Years later Anne learned that her mother had taken Malcolm to have him assessed for dementia by a geriatrician, and he was found to have early signs of dementia. Shirley begged the physician to allow Malcolm to retain his driver's licence. To justify the fact that he was still driving Shirley became a dedicated backseat driver.

The final realization that her father was living with dementia was when Anne got a call from her mother who had just returned from an Alzheimer's support group. She called crying because she just realized at the meeting that Alzheimer's has no cure. At that point she knew that she needed someone to talk to, but initially she pushed back on accepting help from Anne.

After some relatively good years of retired life together, Anne's mom developed pancreatic cancer. Shirley's sister moved in to help her and her sister got to see the level of Malcolm's challenges. She discussed what she observed with Anne. This was a challenging situation because her 79-year-old mother had cancer and her 82-year-old father had Alzheimer's. Luckily, her brother, who had retired, returned home to help out. Shirley died and Anne's brother returned home to Ontario. Anne arranged for someone to help her dad in his home.

Brenda

Brenda is the daughter and primary caregiver of Clifford, who is an 85-year-old African Nova Scotian. When Clifford was 81 his daughter became increasingly concerned about his memory loss and other behaviours. After three tests over a number of years, he was diagnosed with dementia. At the time of the interview he still lived in his own home with Brenda as caregiver with support from homecare services paid for by Veterans Affairs Canada (VAC).

Clifford is one of six children in a family that is not unfamiliar with dementia. His mother had it, as did a sister. He was raised in a small, rural African Nova Scotian community.

Clifford and his wife had three children. His wife died when he was in his late sixties, and he busied himself with activities at the local Legion Hall where he would go most days. Brenda, Clifford's daughter, became his major support and she prepared his evening meal every day. This provided her with the opportunity to monitor him closely without becoming obtrusive. The first thing that Brenda noticed as being odd was that Clifford would line various things up on the windowsill. The first time she became aware of this behaviour he was lining up peach pits and it progressed from there.

He soon began to forget things but not to the extent that Brenda had concerns about him maintaining his independence. Brenda had a house right next to her father's ("forty steps away"), so she was able to follow all his activities carefully. In this period his conversations were typical, but she started to notice that his dates were off or he couldn't relate to dates at all. She remembers the decline as very slow, but when her sister from New Brunswick would visit she would see significant changes, which she pointed out to Brenda.

When Clifford was 81 Brenda began to get concerned about her dad looking after the wood furnace in his home. She also noticed that his dress was becoming more "haphazard." Clifford was still driving to the Legion every day, but one evening he did not come home. Brenda called the Legion and they said that Clifford had left hours ago. They looked for him everywhere and finally he arrived home. He got out of the car and threw his keys. There was no discussion about what happened, but he was clearly scared and not willing to drive again. Brenda then became his chauffeur or travel coordinator as she found people to drive him to his activities.

After three tests over a number of years Clifford was deemed to have dementia. Because of his military service Clifford was entitled to VAC benefits and Brenda contacted them to arrange for homecare services. Homecare workers came four days a week. Clifford did not wander and was not typically up through the night so nighttime care was not a concern. Brenda used a monitoring system between the two houses which helped her to know exactly what was happening in Clifford's home.

Claire

Claire is a 72-year-old currently living in Sydney, Cape Breton. Her mother Florence died six years ago at the age of 92 while in hospital in Halifax where she was "supposed to be taken care of for Alzheimer's disease." At the time of her mother's death, Claire was still working for the federal government, in the department of finance as a policy analyst, on Prince Edward Island. She moved to Cape Breton after retirement because "I had good friends here who lived in Mabou but growing up in a city I decided to come to Sydney." She remembered,

> My father called me to say that mother was having bad memory issues, forgetting things and sometimes expressing frustration and confusion at losing things. He wanted me to go home to deal with her. He was a traditional man who believed that this was women's work. I do have a brother but he lived in another province and was not expected to provide care for Mother.

While still working, Claire said that although she called the family

> once a week on Sundays, I did not visit often, usually at Easter and Christmas and one week a year when I had holidays. I used to travel quite a bit and belonged to several walking groups, so normally went to Europe and other countries while on holiday. I did get along with my parents very well, but was always independent and taught to be so.

Claire said that even though she asked her brother what he thought of their mother's health and that he agreed with her, he said that on their holiday visits and phone calls she seemed "the same as ever — cheerful, always asking what we had been up to and just generally the same as ever."

When Claire returned home for a week, as requested by her father, she did notice that her mother

> seemed distracted and often confused and did seem to have memory issues. I had no intention of leaving my job to care for her so after speaking with my brother and father we agreed that I would hire a

private live-in caregiver for her. The house was a large one with five bedrooms and three bathrooms so there was no issue with space. I approached a local agency in the city and interviewed three different women before choosing one. Although my father was anxious about how this would affect his privacy he agreed it was the best solution at the time.

When Claire hired Grace, she insisted that "she give me bi-weekly updates on Mother's health and she did that. She provided excellent care to my mother and I felt re-assured that she was in good hands. At that point Mother had not seen a doctor nor been diagnosed."

After two years of caring for Florence, Grace suggested that she take her to the family doctor for a checkup as she was concerned that her memory loss and agitation were increasing. At that time and "after extensive tests on her memory, comprehension and understanding, she was diagnosed with Alzheimer's disease. I asked Grace if Mother's care would still be manageable for her and she agreed that it would be, for now, as she phrased it."

Claire talked about the ways in which her mother was a "typical mother,"

My parents had a rigid set of roles. Mother did all the cooking and shopping, she planned and organized all of the family meals, arranged the social calendars for her and Father, took my brother and me to all of our activities as children, made dinners for Father's friends when they came for meetings at the house — all of the typical wifely duties which she seemed happy to undertake. Father was an active volunteer in local business groups like the Halifax Chamber of Commerce and the Downtown Halifax Business Association. He was also a member of the Halifax Club — a private members club for business people. He had few household duties; my brother took care of the garbage and if things needed repair or replacement my father hired workers to do that.

Dale

Dale, in her mid-fifties, shared the story of supporting her friend Peggy who had dementia and died in 2019 at the age of 97. Peggy had cared for her husband David who had Alzheimer's disease and died in 2013 at the age of 97. They married in Montreal in 1949 and both were prominent members of a small town in Kings County.

Dale was profoundly affected by her friend Peggy. Peggy was a mentor to many community activists and Dale treasured the mentoring that Peggy offered her. Dale and Peggy had many common interests and Dale, being the age of Peggy's children, looked up to Peggy for her life experience, her wisdom and her common sense. Dale first met Peggy at a Quaker meeting where she had to interview her in an "icebreaker" exercise. Peggy had just arrived back from a working trip to Romania, where she was working with organizations to help establish democracy in that country. Through the years their friendship solidified. Peggy became Dale's encourager and supporter. "She was one of the few people who could say, 'You're better than this Dale' or 'Get a grip' and I would know she was right, and I would change my attitude."

Dale visited Peggy weekly:

I would take challenges I was facing to her and she would always give sage advice. This relationship helped me, and I think it helped her too. She always knew that I would be by for a visit, and where she lived alone I was a connection to the outside world. Her family was very engaged in her life, but I was the sustained link to her previous work and activism. When you live to be 90 you don't have many friends your own age left so I also helped to fill the gap of missing friends.

As Peggy got into her nineties Dale started to notice that Peggy's memory was slipping but not to the degree that she thought of dementia. Dale said that she thought it was Peggy's age or maybe fatigue that was affecting her.

A couple of days after Peggy had surgery on her eyes (where she had full anesthesia) she had a fall at home and following this she was admitted to long-term care. This was when Dale really started to notice changes in Peggy's mental ability. She was admitted to care for physical reasons, and she was clearly the most mentally competent resident on her floor when she went into care but this began to change. "I felt that I was losing my friend and mentor."

Peggy realized that her mental capacity was changing, and she started sharing the history of her life with Dale.

She wanted me to know everything and I became her confidant. I think the fact that I am a counsellor and understand how to shape a question to get a full story helped in this process. I realized that there are things people want to share with their friends that they may not want to share with their children. I heard a lot about her childhood home in Quebec, her first husband and canoeing on a river where she went to find real peace.

Deanna

Deanna is a 24-year-old honours student at a small university in Kings County. Her grandmother, Riet (known to the family as Oma), is 82 and she was diagnosed with Alzheimer's disease in 2018. Riet now resides in a nursing home in a rural town in the county. Deanna's ancestors first came to Canada during the Netherlands Farm Families Movement after the Second World War, and this heritage still remains strong in the values of the older members of the family, including Riet. Deanna recalled that Oma first started showing symptoms of Alzheimer's disease when she started to

have memory loss. She also got grumpy for no reason and couldn't always focus on what she was doing. She used to be a really strict housekeeper and was always cleaning up, then she didn't seem to care anymore about how clean the house was, and this was so not her usual self. Mom wondered if it was some sort of dementia but Oma being so stubborn, she would not talk about it.

While Riet's family in Nova Scotia were concerned for her health,

eventually one of Mom's brothers, who was visiting from Ontario, suggested that he take Oma to the doctor (he was always her favourite son) and she agreed. That was when they diagnosed the early stages of dementia. Eventually the symptoms got worse and that was when the doctor told Mom that it was likely Alzheimer's.

Prior to her grandmother's diagnosis,

we talked every week on the phone. Sunday was her favourite after she got home from church. Now she doesn't use the phone very much, even though Mom and Dad bought her a cell phone. She can't figure out how to use it, even when the staff help her to put in the numbers.

Deanna played many roles in her grandmother's life. She noted:

My role had been that of the favourite granddaughter to Oma, as I was the only one. She was always so proud of everything I did. She taught me how to cook, especially bake cakes (my favourite), as well she taught me how to knit, milk cows, make butter and cheese (although I never do those things now). She was my best friend for the longest time until she started to forget who I am. This was truly hard for me because even though she would smile at me, she really didn't know who I was. It is such a weird feeling to look at someone you love and know they love you and not have them recognize you. I know it is very hard on Mom too. She is one of three siblings, and her brothers both live in Ontario, so since the pandemic she can't visit or help out with Oma.

Deb and Cathy

Deb is 58 and Cathy is 61. They have been partners for thirty-two years and were among the first lesbians to marry in Nova Scotia. Deb's family originates from Europe and she is Caucasian while Cathy is African Nova Scotian and her family goes back "a really long way to the days of slavery." Each of them is the primary caregiver for one of their parents. Deb's mother, Lucy, is 84 and was diagnosed with dementia four years ago. Cathy's father, Ernie, who is 89, was diagnosed with dementia four years ago, just a year after her mother died of cancer. They all live in Nova Scotia; Lucy, Deb and Cathy live in a large suburb outside of a major city. Ernie lives in a predominantly African Canadian community in the same city.

Deb said that she first noticed changes in her mom's behaviour when they used to get together to play cards and her mom would forget what she was playing. As well, she started forgetting to pick up groceries and clean the house.

Mom was also such a tidy person, neurotically you might say. Then she started to let the house go and also her appearance. She was always so fussy about the way she looked and then she sort of forgot to brush her hair, that sort of thing. As she got worse — and my sisters noticed too when they talked to her on the phone — I took her to our doctor and she diagnosed her with dementia but she said that without further tests she couldn't say which type. Mom wasn't happy about having more tests so we didn't go for that. The doctor referred Mom to the Home Care people and they assessed her and said she could have a CCA come into the house twice a day to check on her, at least for now.

Cathy said that after her mom died her dad

sort of fell apart. He was often confused, kept forgetting things and just wasn't himself. I figured it was because he was grieving and I talked to the pastor about it and she came to the house to talk with him. She agreed that he seemed more than sad and grieving and suggested I talk to our doctor about it. He wasn't up for that and said he was scared after what happened to Mom and her getting diagnosed with cancer when she went to see a doctor. So, I left it for a while. Then he had a really bad case of pneumonia and he had to go for tests, so we got him to see the geriatric specialist who was there that day and he said Dad had dementia. It was a real shock because Dad has always been the one in charge of everything. Suddenly I had to be, and I wasn't sure I could do that. Fortunately for us in some ways, by then Deb's mom had been diagnosed so we were able to help each other out.

Diane

Diane is 63 and she lives in a small town in Kings County. Her father Joseph was first diagnosed with dementia in 2014 and later died in a nursing home in that county two years ago at the age of 81. As well as caring for her father, Diane concurrently cared for her mother prior to her death from kidney disease.

Joseph developed the early signs of dementia while he was caring for his wife. Diane recalls that she did not notice any signs of dementia in her dad until six years ago when her parents moved to NS. "In retrospect there were signs well before, but we [family] did not consider dementia. Perhaps because there was no history of dementia in our family, or that we more focused on my mother and her health issues."

We scheduled a doctor's appointment for an assessment. Dad was diagnosed with dementia in October of 2014. He was 81-years-old. I did not feel particularly distressed in the beginning as Dad continued to be pleasant, positive and easygoing.

Dad was Mom's support person for home hemodialysis which he became less capable of. He stopped driving and being able to run errands to the grocery store in 2017. My role did not ,change significantly when I started helping because I was always the "caregiver" (nurse) in the family. However, I did have to help with Dad's personal care, which was a new role.

Trying to determine how to best "help" was often difficult. You cannot develop a routine or schedule with dementia; you have to be able to relinquish any sense of control and learn to just "go with the flow." The situation with Alzheimer's is always fluid; sometimes the person may be lucid, others not. You have to be able to deal with each situation as it comes up.

Donalda

Donalda is a 46-year-old African Nova Scotian woman who lives in a "mainly Black community just outside of Halifax." She lives with her husband, Brandon, and two of her three children, both teenagers. Two years ago, her mother-in-law, Grace, moved in with the family after being diagnosed with Alzheimer's disease. Donalda worked as a receptionist in a dental practice but when her mother-in-law moved in she had to quit her job to take care of her. Brandon is still working as a labourer and one of their sons Jessie, who is 18, works for an IT company part time while also attending university. Her other son who lives at home, Jonathon, is 16 and he is still in high school. Donalda's daughter, Katrina, is at university in another province and is 20.

Prior to being diagnosed with Alzheimer's, Grace worked as a cashier in a grocery store part time while she took care of her husband, Tyrone, who died of small cell prostate cancer six months after his diagnosis.

The family first noticed that Grace was "behaving different" when she no longer wanted to sing in the church choir,

> *something she had loved to do since she was a small child. We figured it was because she missed Tyrone and was still grieving, but we thought that would have been when she most wanted to go to church and sing the Lord's praises for all the other things she had in her life.*

As well as changes in her behaviour Donalda also noticed that Grace was getting forgetful and "sometimes mixed up her days. When we tried to talk to her about it, she would always tell us to mind our own business and she would be cranky. This wasn't like her and again we just thought it was the grief talking." Donalda spoke with the minister of their local church to ask if she would talk to Grace about these matters, in case it was more than grief. When the minister got back to the family she told them that Grace was feeling very scared about forgetting things, especially some of the words of the hymns she had sung since a child, and that was why she didn't want to go to church any more. The minister suggested that the family have a talk with Grace's doctor about her memory problems and see what he felt about it. Initially Grace was very reluctant to go to him, but when Brandon offered to go with her, she agreed. "The doctor suggested that Grace go for memory tests, saying that the problems might be related to the blood pressure pills she was on, and he wanted to rule them out."

Brandon and Donalda accompanied Grace to the memory clinic, where they gave her a series of tests aimed at "testing her memory and her comprehension." The results indicated that Grace was "probably in the early stages of Alzheimer's and they recommended some memory exercises for her to do with us, as well as asking her doctor for medication, not to cure the illness but to hopefully keep it at bay."

As Alzheimer's progressed and Grace became more confused and angry at her memory loss, after "a lot and lot of talks about it and the kids not being happy about having her in the home," the family agreed that Grace should move in with them. Brandon does have two brothers, but both live in Ontario and neither wanted their mother living with them. Donalda said, "We really didn't have no choice; we didn't want her in no home for old people and we knew she would be best with her own kind."

Grace was a

> real mother to her boys. She loved them so much and was always good to them. Education was important to her and she wanted them to do well in life. She made some of their clothes when they were little. She was a good cook and always had them looking clean and smart. She was a good mother-in-law to me, always helping us out when she could. When we decided that we wanted to live in our own house, rather than keep renting, she loaned us some money for a down payment even though they didn't have much at the time. Their kids were everything to them. Grace is very religious, and she loves the Lord. She prayed every day and tried to get my kids to as well, but they are typical young folk — don't believe no more but do come to church if I asks them to. She used to be a real

force in the church, not just in the choir but also helping with the school breakfast program, doing some outreach work with folk whose loved ones had passed on, and generally just doing whatever needed to be done there.

As well as her family responsibilities and her work for the church, Grace was

highly involved in the local community. If something needed to be done here, they always called her to help out. She and Tyrone helped build a community playground for local children and when we had family outings and events, she always made her beans and corn bread muffins that were a real treat. Everyone around here loves her and they sure do miss seeing her around.

Edith

Edith is an 86-year-old woman who lives in a small town in Kings County, Nova Scotia. Her husband, Tom, was 83 when he died of Alzheimer's in a nursing home three years ago. Edith now lives with her daughter and husband in a house they renovated after she sold the one she and Tom lived in because "the house became too much for me on my own. We were very sad to leave it as it had been my family home for over forty years." Edith had been married before and her husband died of cancer at the age of 46; at that time two of her three children lived at home and she became a single parent. Edith first met Tom at a "card game held at a local church. They had card games and potluck suppers and I often went with friends. A very good friend introduced us and we went from there, going out for lunches and dinners and getting to know each other better." A year after they met, Tom proposed to Edith and she accepted. She recalls his proposal: "We went to a local restaurant for my birthday supper and he actually got down on one knee — can you imagine in front of everyone — and asked me to marry him. How could I refuse such a romantic offer?" After they married, Tom gave up his rented apartment and moved into Edith's house.

From her first marriage Edith had three children: two daughters (one with whom she now lives and the other lives in the United States) and a son (who lives in British Columbia). Edith has three grandchildren as well as three great-grandchildren. Two of them live close by, and the other lives in Boston. Edith and Tom were married for twenty-six years. Before she retired, Edith worked as a high school administrator. Tom worked in construction for a local company.

Edith first noticed Tom's behaviour change when he

started to get forgetful. He used to love to go fishing after he retired and sometimes he would call me and ask me how he could get home. He would forget where he lived. We had one of the phones where you could just hit "home" and the GPS would give you instructions, so I would tell him to do that. It wasn't so bad when he went with friends because they would drive, but when he was on his own I was so worried about him.

As well as forgetting how to get home, Tom also had other memory issues.

He loved to do the cryptic crosswords in the newspaper and then he stopped; he said he couldn't remember the formulas he had created to solve the puzzles. He did switch to the regular crosswords but couldn't remember those words either. He said it was because he was having "senior moments" and there was nothing to worry about.

In spite of her concerns, Tom refused to go to see his doctor. "He had this thing about doctors, hospitals and clinics and kept refusing to go. He said there was nothing wrong with him and I was making a fuss about nothing." Edith talked to her daughter Liz about her concerns and together they finally talked Tom into going to see a doctor. "I told him to do it for me because I was worried about him and that it was making me sick." When they saw their family doctor he sent Tom for various tests and as a result he was diagnosed with "probable Alzheimer's disease." Tom was placed on medications for the disease as well as for anxiety which resulted after his diagnosis.

He was so anxious all the time. The doctor told him he couldn't drive anymore and that really upset him. He was one of those men who thought that the man in the family should do the driving, even though I can drive, and I just went along with it. It really bothered him that there were things he couldn't do anymore and he felt very badly with me having to do them.

On some occasions Tom would still try to do some of his previous activities but with serious consequences.

> *It was always his job to take out the garbage and I had to do it because he would forget where to put it or wander up the road. One time, while I was in the shower, he just took it out (we kept the containers outside on the porch) and he fell and really hurt himself. It was winter and he missed the steps and went down face first. He had to have stitches to his face; he had such a bad cut.*

On another occasion,

> *it was yard sale Saturday and I was taking out stuff to the curbside that we didn't need. The next thing I know he is bringing out a chair from the kitchen to put out. He dropped it on his foot and was in a lot of pain. When I tried to explain to him that we weren't selling it, he just couldn't understand why I was putting out some stuff and not everything.*

Tom was 76 when he was diagnosed with Alzheimer's disease and Edith said "that it came on suddenly and he deteriorated really fast."
The roles which Tom played in their family were

> *typical male ones. He did most of the driving, he took care of the finances, mowed the lawn and did the garbage. It wasn't that he couldn't or wouldn't do housework or laundry and that sort of thing, and he had to when I broke my wrist one time, but he preferred it if I did these things. He changed the oil in the car and the windshield washer fluid and wipers. He changed the oil in the ride-on mower too. After he retired he did sometimes come with me to do the groceries and go to the liquor store but he wasn't fond of shopping much.*

As well as these domestic roles, Tom was also a

> *very good dad. When they were little he liked to give them their baths at night and we shared doing the bedtime stories. Of course, being an avid fisherman, he taught them all how to fish and he even coached soccer for a few years, until they all got interested in hockey instead and he couldn't coach that.*

Edith said that Tom was also her

> *best friend and a good listener, not just to me but also the kids. If we had things we couldn't work out, we could always talk to him*

and he was great at seeing the different sides of a problem. It was him who liked to have family dinners on Sundays with Liz and her brood, even though they weren't blood relations to him. I was always the one who remembered birthdays and organized the Christmas and Easter cards, and he never bought the presents or any of those things. He was happy for me to be in charge then.

Faye

Faye married Bob knowing that he had early signs of dementia. She loved him and wanted to provide the care he needed while she was able. Bob was eventually admitted to a nursing home, but Faye indicated that she did not regret having the time that she and Bob shared.

Faye lives in a small Nova Scotia town. Unbeknownst to her, when Faye first met Bob he had already been diagnosed with dementia. In spite of this he could, with some help, manage to live independently, make his own meals, keep track of his schedule and maintain an active social life. He stuck to a regime he established for himself that involved walking every day. This is where Faye saw him regularly. They also bumped into each other at church and arts events.

Bob's wife of sixty-two years had died, and Faye had recently lost her husband. Bob and Faye struck up a friendship that involved eating and participating in social activities together. She noted that in their first year of friendship he was very rational and could share wonderful stories from his past. What she started to notice is the stories got recycled and she would hear them again and again. She invited him to speak to a local women's group about a recent trip to Europe and his presentation was very awkward and poorly constructed. She called Bob's daughter and asked her about this. This was the first time she learned about Bob's dementia.

The effects of the dementia became more obvious as time progressed. One time Bob was driving to a family event. Faye called his attention to the fact that he had turned the wrong way and were on a major highway, so he proceeded to make a U-turn. They were both terrified and he quietly relinquished the driver's seat to Faye. She did most of the driving after that.

Faye wanted to care for him as it was becoming obvious that he would need care. One day while she had her head in the fridge looking for something for lunch, Bob proposed. She did not hesitate to say "yes." They signed a pre-nuptial agreement, found a minister who knew the situation and were married at a family cottage. Bob moved into Faye's home and accepted it as his own.

Ginger

Ginger said that her mother, Sally, is a residential school survivor and her early life experiences led to life-long harmful involvement with alcohol. It was difficult for the family to recognize the dementia as "we never really knew if [what we observed] was the effects of dementia or the alcohol."

Jan

Jan's interview took place in the courtyard of a retirement living residence where she lives in a small community in Kings County. She is a retired university professor who was diagnosed five years ago with the early stages of mixed dementia, which she said is a "combination of Alzheimer's disease and vascular dementia." Jan is 84 years old. She did not initially meet our criteria as a caregiver for a person with dementia, but when she heard about our research she asked to be a part of it, and we agreed that her perspective could add yet another set of experiences to this timely topic. When we met for the interview, Jan brought along a folder with information and notes she had been taking of her journey through the disease because she was concerned that her memories would not always be accurate. Jan has a unique perspective on noticing dementia as she is caring for herself in a supportive care environment while living with the condition. Jan relates, "Not only do I experience memory problems but I also have trouble with problem solving, confusion and other ones too." As well as this condition, Jan also experiences dizziness and loss of balance, which her family doctor suggested was a result of "the anxiety and depression I was feeling when I started to have memory loss and confusion." Jan was diagnosed after she was having issues with some of the above symptoms as well as

> remembering things like names, faces and words and sometimes what days of the week it was. Some days are still like that, so I come and go in terms of memory. I can remember what I did when I was a child, but usually not what I had for breakfast that morning.

Jan said the worst losses were "when I couldn't remember the names of my plants. I had a lovely garden and after I retired, I spent as much time there as I could. When people would admire the flowers and ask me what they were I could always tell them, and losing that ability was really frightening." As a result of these symptoms Jan decided to sell her home, which is in the same town as she lives now, even though

> it really broke my heart to give up the house. But, I knew I couldn't manage on my own anymore and I knew other people who lived here in the assisted care facility, so decided it was as good a place as any to live and I get my meals and some help with cleaning and medications as well. If I am being totally honest too, I was lonely. I have lived alone for a long time, since Timothy [her son] went off to film school in LA, and I was very social. But with the balance issues and the depression I didn't want to go out and I wasn't seeing people the way I used to.

Jan said that when she talked to her doctor, he told her that people who live alone are harder to diagnose because "we don't have other people to observe and confirm our losses. That made sense to me." Jan moved to her present location four and a half years ago.

Janet

Janet is one of two children and the only daughter of Judy. Janet and Judy live close to one another in Halifax, and while providing increasing levels of support, Janet continues to encourage Judy's independence. As early as age 60 Janet noticed that Judy was forgetting things. She was very social but those around her also noticed that she repeated the same story. She had memory tests and assessments and was diagnosed with late-onset Attention Deficit Hyperactivity Disorder (ADHD). Janet never believed this diagnosis as Judy had trouble remembering things, but she was always able to focus. Judy was also diagnosed with depression, which was treated with medication.

It would not have surprised anyone that Judy had Alzheimer's disease. Her father had it and her mother volunteered at the Alzheimer Society of Nova Scotia and understood the disease well. In spite of the expectation that at some point Judy would be diagnosed with Alzheimer's disease, it took a decade of persistent visits to physicians and specialists before they finally heard what her daughter expected all along.

At the age of 72 Judy's score on memory tests reached the point that her physician deemed she had dementia. It was interesting for Janet to see what the tests measured because her mother still had excellent long-term memory and she remained creative, but she had trouble remembering things that happened very recently and she could not always determine the order in which things should happen.

At a certain point Judy was required to move. Janet felt that Judy was not yet ready for long-term care, but she would need daily support and that would require her to be in close proximity to Janet. She moved into an apartment a block away from Janet.

Janet commented on packing for this move. She and her brother would pack boxes according to the room in which they would be unpacked. Her mother would re-pack them in what appeared to be a totally random manner. There would be small pockets of things that were completely unrelated all packed together. "I realized," said Janet, "how her condition results in a mind that functions in a seemingly random manner."

As time progressed Janet started to assume increasing levels of responsibility for Judy's finances and the general coordination of her life — groceries, transportation, problems with technology and communication with family. Judy returned to the US to visit her mother every year and as her memory became more problematic Janet travelled with her. One year Janet purchased tickets for the flight to the US but before she and her mother left, Judy's mother died. Janet explained this to her mother, but Judy believed that they had originally purchased the tickets to attend the memorial service and appeared to be unaffected by the fact that her mother had died. It was at this point that Janet realized that her mother was losing touch with her former self.

Jeff

Jeff is "in his sixties" and lives "just outside Halifax" with his mother Stella who is 84 years old. She was diagnosed with Alzheimer's four years ago. Jeff is a retired optometry assistant, and his mother did not work outside of the home. Jeff said that his mother started to

> go wobbly in her brain, just like her mom did. Granny Nelly we called her — but then we just thought it was due to old age. Her husband Stan was the same, and we just thought with him it was because he had been in the war. I wonder sometimes if older people had Alzheimer's then, but we just didn't know how to test them for it, or what to call it.

When pressed for more information about Stella exhibiting "wobbly" behaviours Jeff said that she "seemed to be forgetting things — names of things and people, stuff we would normally buy at the grocery store, those everyday types of things. She was confused sometimes too and just seemed not her usual cheery self." Jeff is an only child and his father Kenny died thirty years ago, "so then there was just Mom living on her own. I lived with my partner Steve then but when he died of non-Hodgkin's related disease related to HIV, I decided to move in with Mom."

Part of Stella's confusion, according to Jeff, is that

> she doesn't always know who I am. I could be me, or our neighbour Chris next door, or her brother Dave who died years ago. When I wake up in the mornings I often think "Who will I be today?" I always wanted to be an actor but not on this stage! There's just so many roles I could play in her mind, so I don't always know who I am either. It's a bit schizophrenic. The other day when I came in from putting the garbage in the shed she asked me when I was coming to visit. I said, "When who is coming to visit?" She said "Jeff." I said, "I am Jeff" and she said to me, "You can't be. He's much better looking" — sheesh what a way to cheer a guy up. You have to laugh, don't you; otherwise you would weep and not stop.

When he first noticed changes in Stella's behaviour, Jeff said that he was

> scared that she was going down the same road as her parents, but I kept dismissing those thoughts because I didn't want to be negative. She seemed mostly the same as ever and it didn't seem to bother her that she forgot things now and then. More now than then of course. In the beginning I didn't do anything about it but then I was talking to one of the ophthalmologists in the clinic and she said her mom had similar issues so I should probably have a chat with our doctor. I knew Mom wouldn't agree to that so I called the office and explained my worries to the receptionist there and she said they would call and say that Mom was due for a checkup. She also has diabetes and they check that out regularly, so that seemed like a good solution.

After a series of tests that their doctor ordered, Stella was diagnosed with the "beginning stages of Alzheimer's." At that time, Stella refused to believe it and said she was just having "the usual old age problems with her memory." According to Jeff, even when lucid she still refuses to acknowledge that she has the disease.

Jeff said that his mother always "took great care of me, being an only child and all that. I was probably spoiled rotten. Things could be tense between us sometimes because she could be very bossy, but we mostly got along well, especially after Dad died and there was just the two of us rubbing along together as a family. Stella was an

> excellent cook. She could bake anything you wanted. She always made my birthday cakes by hand; she would never buy a cake from a store. She made some of my clothes when I was little. I wore pink shirts before they became the "in" thing. She did all the cooking, cleaning and shopping in the family, was the one who kept all the books and she had lists of whose birthdays were when, even my friends at school, so we could always send cards. She was the one who made the gifts to give teachers at Christmas and she kept everything in the family running like clockwork.

Jeff said he was a

> good son to them both. I always kept in touch. When Steve and me were together we either had them, and then her, for Sunday brunch or we took them out or went to their house. We took them out for their birthdays and anniversaries and sometimes drove them for day trips on a Sunday.

Now Jeff

> does everything that needs be done. I still take her for Sunday drives; she loves that even though she never remembers where we are going anymore and keeps asking me where we are now. I wake her up, help her have a wash and get dressed. On good days we fight about my choices of clothes for her to wear, otherwise she couldn't care less, but she won't spend a day in her nightdress. I do the errands and clean the house, do the laundry and iron now and then. When she's "up" I do her hair colour. She always hated having white hair, so I buy dye and colour her hair. It is a lot of work, but she is my mom, and that's what you do, isn't it?

John

John lives in HRM. He and his wife, Sandy, both grew up in Nova Scotia and met in high school. After they each moved away from their hometown and married others, they met again in later life and after the death of a spouse and a divorce, they got married. John is 78 and Sandy is 80. Four years ago John noticed that Sandy was starting to experience "memory lapses" where she would forget the days of the week and routine things like doing the laundry and shopping for food. John said, "Sandy was very routine oriented so every week she did the same things on the same days and then it seemed like she was just disorganized." He asked her several times if she realized that she was forgetting things and she said that she was just "having senior moments."

John said that as his wife's symptoms continued, he felt "very scared that she might be getting the Alzheimer's because we have friends who have, and she was starting to go that way." As Sandy's memory loss increased, she also became agitated when John questioned her about it. He suggested that they go together for a memory test. "I thought if I said I was getting forgetful too and wanted to get it checked out that we could go together, and it wouldn't be all about her."

They did go together for a memory test and were told that indeed Sandy did have acute memory loss and should see a GP. John remembers that "Sandy was really mad about that and said she was just having an off day. I lied and said that I hadn't done well on the tests either so we should go together to see our family doctor." After they saw their family doctor, she did suggest that Sandy "showed signs of dementia" and suggested that they keep an eye on her symptoms in case they increased. The doctor also suggested that they participate in a clinical trial research program being held in various locations across the province to test new medications for the disease. John said that the program is very time consuming:

> *Once a week we go to Halifax where they start with a bunch of questions they ask her, then she has an infusion of the medicine or the placebo — we don't know which — that takes about an hour. After that they monitor her blood pressure and heart rate and other stuff for another two hours, I suppose to see if she has side effects. Then after a lunch break they ask me a bunch of questions about what we did yesterday, then they ask her the same questions, then we all talk about what she remembers of what happened yesterday.*

He said further that the process "lasts about eight hours and after we get home we are both really tired." John said that expenses such as travel and meals are covered by the program. But "even though it doesn't cost us anything, it is very time consuming and just makes a lot more work for me."

Kelli

Kelli used to live in Mahone Bay, Nova Scotia, but moved to Ontario to be closer to her daughter and grandson after her mother died. She is 72 and a retired nurse. Her mother, Grace, "had been diagnosed with bipolar disorder in her late twenties. As a result of her bipolar disorder and diabetes, which she also had as a younger woman, she experienced several miscarriages until I was born, and she had no other children after me." She also had two heart attacks in her early eighties, so the eventual diagnosis of Alzheimer's disease was not unexpected. Grace died three years ago at the age of 93 in a nursing home close to their home.

Grace was widowed in her sixties when her husband died of a stroke. Before her hospitalization and then death, she lived in Lunenburg, where she also worked as a clerk in a grocery store before and after her husband's death.

Kelli said that her mother was always

having mood swings and could get very low with depression. So, when she also started to have memory problems, I just assumed it was to do with that. We talked every day on the phone, and I visited every other weekend or sometimes in the week depending on my shifts at the hospital. I worked on the psych ward, so I was familiar with some of the symptoms of different types of dementia and did wonder if that was what was going on.

Kelli said that normally in their interactions

Mom was her usual self, so it was kinda hard to tell what was going on with her, but I did notice that her memory was getting really bad and that was when I suggested she go for some tests. Initially she did well, but after about six months we went again and she was much worse, so they recommended more tests and that's when we found out it was Alzheimer's.

Grace was

somewhere in her late seventies when she got the diagnosis. At first

she refused to accept it, but then when it was clear she couldn't man-
age on her own — she kept forgetting to turn off the kettle, or the
stove, or feed the cat — then she agreed to have Home Care come in.

While Grace was doing well on her own with home support services daily, Kelli was becoming more concerned about her health and well-being, especially as Grace was

becoming more and more depressed at the things she couldn't do
anymore. She didn't like the way they [the Home Care staff] did the
dishes, or did the laundry and ironing and she said they put things
away in the wrong places, and she couldn't find anything. Every
day when I called or saw her, she would do nothing but complain
about them, so I looked into having her go into a private care home.

Kelli said that after putting her mother's name down on a waiting list, she finally found a place which would take her. It was a

nursing home in my community, so that I could check in on her
and make sure she was being well taken care of. Initially she really
hated it, but eventually she seemed to almost like being there and
the staff were kind and caring. It wasn't perfect by any means; there
weren't enough staff and the dementia wing was a nightmare. It
wasn't always clean, and some residents sat in their own mess for
a long time before they were changed.

Kelli said that when she decided to have her mother placed in a care facility she

thought long and hard about it. I felt very badly that I didn't want
her in my home and I didn't want to stop working to take care of
her. I really experienced a tremendous amount of guilt over my
decision, but I knew that it wouldn't work for her to live with me.

As Grace's condition worsened,

she was getting argumentative with the other residents and staff.
She was in adult diapers and kept taking them off and accidentally
peed in the public places, which meant they had to clean up all the
time, and she started yelling at people. The administrator called
me to say that she was upsetting the other residents and that she

needed more care than they could provide, and she needed to be in either a hospital or a different type of nursing home.

As well as causing distress to the staff and other residents of the nursing home, Grace was also causing a

great deal of stress for me. I had purchased a cell phone for her and only put in my number and my daughter's so that she could call at any time. She used to phone me in the middle of the night to tell me that the staff had stolen her babies, or she would say that she had no clothes because they had been taken by other residents. When I would try to comfort her and tell her that the babies died before they were born, she would tell me that I was lying. It was absolutely heartbreaking to go through this night after night. I knew she wasn't in her right mind, but it still hurt me so much. I used to wish that she would just die, so she wouldn't have to suffer so much pain and loss; then of course when she did die, I blamed myself for wishing it to be.

While Kelli was contemplating her options, Grace "fell and broke her hip, so then the decision was out of my hands and she had to be hospitalized." While in the hospital Grace was

really out of it most of the time, she didn't know why she was there, who anybody was and why they were doing things to her, she didn't know me and would get so angry at being kept in there. She kept asking me where Dick was (her husband) and why he wasn't coming to take her home and where all her babies were. I never realized what impact the miscarriages must have had on her because it was something she hardly ever talked about. It was the most difficult experience of my life to go through all of this. I never saw her happy at anything and the hospital staff seemed to lose patience with her a lot. As a nurse, I appreciate how difficult their work is and especially with these types of patients, they are all overworked and have no time to spend with any particular person, but they should have changed her bedding more often, made sure she ate and kept her clean. Some days the food from breakfast would be sitting there uneaten and the room would stink. When they called me to say she had gone, my first feeling was relief, for her and for me, what kind of daughter thinks that?

Laura

Laura and Jack are in their late sixties. This is the second marriage for each of them and they have been together for thirty years. They moved to a small Nova Scotia town following Jack's retirement. About three years ago Jack was diagnosed with Parkinson's disease. His diagnosis of dementia is connected to his cognitive impairment associated with Parkinson's. This is Laura's second encounter with the disease as it claimed her father's life.

Laura did not think her story was relevant to a dementia collection because her husband has been diagnosed as having Parkinson's-related "cognitive impairments." The changes that prompted the assessment of Jack for dementia were difficulty in finding the right words to communicate, reduced ability to organize, plan, reason, or solve problems and difficulty handling complex tasks. She also noted general apathy which required her to organize his daily activities. If left on his own Jack was happy to spend hours playing cards on the computer.

Jack had been a highly motivated individual. He loved to hike, run and restore houses. He had a lifetime career with a large corporation and did very well. Together they raised four children and were now grandparents.

As Laura took on more of the planning functions in their lives — step-by-step planning of house restorations, trips and finances — she was convinced that Jack was developing dementia. This would not be uncommon given that a large number of people with Parkinson's disease develop dementia.

Jack went through the testing and the physicians said that there was no evidence of dementia. As they shared the results of the tests, Laura reported that she kept thinking, "Are you reporting on Jack because I think you have someone else's results." Finally, they said that there was some cognitive decline but no dementia. "What the hell does that mean?" she thought. She asked the physicians for a description of the line between cognitive decline and dementia and she got no clear answer. She has come to believe that while physicians may be helpful in addressing the motor challenges of Parkinson's disease they really have less insight into the cognitive effects of the disease.

Ling

Ling and her husband, Walter, live in Halifax Regional Municipality, where they own and operate a traditional Chinese medical clinic. They are the sole caregivers of their mother/mother-in-law Gao (who Ling calls Yuemu, which is the name she would be called in China). Gao has been diagnosed with the early stages of Alzheimer's disease. She lives at home with Ling and Walter. They moved to Nova Scotia from Richmond, British Columbia, three years ago when Ling and Walter's son Thomas "came to the Halifax Infirmary to do a medical residency. He is now working as a doctor in the Victoria General Hospital." Ling did not provide her age, nor those of her husband and mother-in-law as she did not feel the information was relevant to the interview.

Ling said that Gao was

> *very reluctant to leave Richmond, where she had many friends and good neighbours. She would go to the community centre almost every day, or go to the market to buy food and play Mah-jongg with her friends. Here in Halifax there are no places to go or have Chinese friends and neighbours, so she is very unhappy here.*

Walter is "the only son" and this is of great importance where the couple is from in China. "In the province in China where we lived, family is the most important thing, so she had to come and be with us as we are all here now." Walter has one sister, but she lives in China and is not able to provide active care to their mother.

Gao was diagnosed with Alzheimer's after she

> *had a bad fall down the stairs in the house from her room. An ambulance had to come to take her to the hospital and when she was there we told them she was being confused sometimes and forgetful and was having delusions. We thought it was because she had an imbalance between her Yin and Yang. In China we believe that dementias are a normal part of growing old and they are the fate of all older people.*

Ling suggested that as people grow old, the

> *duality of their lives can be altered so that the energies of Yin and Yang become more diffused. Like the seasons, as we grow old, we go into a winter like phase of life where we rest and relax. We do not fight aging as they do here in the West. We accept it as a normal part of life and death. In China we treat Alzheimer's disease and dementias with special traditional Chinese herbal medicines*

and last year a new drug was created in China to help people with
these maladies.

While in the hospital after the fall, Gao had various tests which determined that she was "depressed, had diabetes and had the early stages of
Alzheimer's disease." Ling said that they did not know about Gao's diabetes
and said that it is likely due

> *to the lack of Chinese food availability in Halifax. In Richmond,*
> *where Chinese people are the majority, there are very many mar-*
> *kets which sell all of the Chinese products we are used to: the salt*
> *fish, the vegetables, barbecued pork, live chickens and many other*
> *things. Here in Halifax there are some stores which sell Chinese*
> *food, but they are not as fresh as in Richmond and not as full of*
> *nutrients. Here when we buy fish, they have no head or tails and*
> *the chickens in the stores have no feet or heads. We use these parts*
> *for soups. Here we are very few Chinese people, so it is hard to find*
> *good food that we are used to.*

Ling said that the hospital had suggested that the family add Gao's
name to the nursing home list so that she could be relocated to one in
their area, but the family refused because in China

> *care of the old is the family's responsibility and we take care of them*
> *at home. We didn't think she would be happy in a nursing home*
> *where they don't know how to cook the foods we eat and how to*
> *take care of her needs. We didn't want her to be the only Chinese*
> *one there either and her English is not very good.*

In their home Gao is the main

> *housekeeper and cook. She keeps the house clean and does most of*
> *the cooking. We are both at work for most of the days and she is*
> *happy to stay home and do these things. She mends and washes the*
> *clothes; she irons them and hangs them in the closets. She also keeps*
> *the shoes clean and shiny. We rely on her to help in these ways as*
> *we are busy working to bring in the money. Once a week I used to*
> *take her to Spencer House [a community centre in Halifax] where*
> *they offered Mah-jongg for some of the older citizens, but now we*
> *cannot go anymore because there is the virus. I know she is lonely*

*at home by herself. In China we feel that it is very important that
our elders feel useful and are able to contribute to the family. Even
when they are frail, they can do some things. I used to take her to
buy the shopping but she didn't really enjoy it. In Richmond and at
home when we shop we go to the markets and we meet people we
know; here people are not as friendly and Gao is not used to the
types of food in the shops here. Because her English is not good she
does not know how to ask for things in the stores she cannot find.
We have met some other Chinese families, but she is not comfortable with them.*

So far, Gao's roles have not had to change as a result of the Alzheimer's disease. She does sometimes

*forget to do things but I use the telephone to check with her every
day while at work and remind her of what to do. We don't expect
everything to be as it was because of the dementia. We are able to use
the acupuncture to help her feel better and she is comfortable with
that. As well, we have Chinese herbs which help with the balance
between the Yin and Yang. We take good care of her, better than
she would have if in a nursing home. We order things from China
and also from Richmond when we cannot find certain things here.*

Loree

Loree, in her mid-sixties, supported her dad, Robert, who was diagnosed with dementia and lived close by in rural Nova Scotia. She reflects on her role as the daughter of someone who lived on their own with dementia, developed a new relationship while living with increasing cognitive challenges and was eventually admitted to a long-term care facility where he died.

Robert and his wife moved to Nova Scotia following retirement from their respective careers, and they built a house that they could age in — everything on the main floor, wheelchair accessibility and a basement apartment for a potential caregiver.

*My mother saw changes in my father in his late seventies. She com-
pensated for these changes but brought them to our attention. My
first role in my father's dance with dementia was that of a skeptic or
an outright denier. I thought that since her retirement my mother*

was just seeing my father for what he always was — a brilliant but somewhat absent-minded fellow who never was particularly competent with household tasks. My father continued to be an engaging conversationalist and a good guest preacher and writer. He loved entertaining, travelling and finding interesting ways to engage with his children and grandchildren.

My mother had breast cancer. The first experience of cancer was in her fifties. Breast cancer disrupted her life again in her early seventies and finally came to stay in her eighties. My mother insisted in her eighties that she was not doing battle with the disease — she was simply going to live with it and accomplish all she could in spite of it. My father was her primary caregiver. She organized this role with routines, lists and notes. When he mixed things up my mother saw this as evidence of his dementia; I saw it as the strain of caregiving.

My mother finally raised her concerns about my father's cognitive challenges with the family physician. He was concerned enough to put my dad on medication, but Dad continued with all his roles so no one really saw anything that could not be explained away. As my brother said in hindsight, "Even when he was failing he was still the smartest person in the room." My first realization that maybe my mother was right came on the last service Dad held as interim minister at a local church. My twin grandchildren were to receive a "blessing" (their parents not adhering to some of our other faith rituals, this was a good compromise). My father took each child in his arms and shared their names with the congregation. In each case the name was wrong. My heart sank as I realized for the first time that my mother was right — Dad's cognitive skills were declining. I became a believer. I increased my visits and looked for ways to be more supportive to my mother.

My mother died when Dad was in his mid-eighties. They were still living in their home and with Dad's care, family visits and support from [the] VON and paid caregivers, Mom was able to die at home. From years of living with my mother's lists and routines Dad was able to establish a regimen that supported him to live a life of independence in spite of his cognitive decline. He called people, walked, attended community events, gardened, connected with people online and even wiggled his way back into preaching. During this period, I took on the role of monitor. I began to meet with him regularly. I watched what he was doing, wearing, eating and saying in an attempt to keep him safe and happy.

One day I noticed that he had a large box in his front hall. I asked him about it, and he informed me that it was full of books. On closer inspection I found that it contained hundreds of copies of a book that my mother had written and self-published, as well as a book that he had written decades ago. As a way to continue in their role as authors Dad had approached an American firm to publish the books and he was part of the distribution process. I asked to see the correspondence regarding this purchase and found that the firm had promised to print and market the books for a ridiculously high price that my father had paid. He knew that he had got in over his head and did not know how to get out. It was sad to see his hard earned dollars be used to line the pockets of unscrupulous people who clearly preyed on those who were unable to look after their own best interests. I had power of attorney and I realized that it was time to become co-decision maker in order to help my father make better decisions. I also began to look after all his finances, leaving him enough in his account to do what he wanted and needed to do.

My father became very popular with the ladies in town and was frequently invited out for dinner or to other activities. He called these "not a date." One woman became a particular favourite, and he began spending more time with her. I knew this woman and I trusted her judgment, so I backed off a bit on monitoring my dad. Knowing that he had a consistent relationship, and I could be alerted if there were issues, my husband and I went to Florida for a couple of weeks. During this time, we arranged for Dad to visit us. It was there that I realized the degree of his challenges — both physical and cognitive. He was helpful, kind and friendly but I realized that he could not tell time and he was not able to plan. Every morning he packed his bag to go home and part way through the day he would get ready for bed. He left Florida before we did and I made a plan — he would not be preaching, driving or living alone. I assumed the role of the enforcer.

Marion

Marion is an 86-year-old married woman and a retired secretary living in HRM with her 89-year-old husband, Dick, who is a retired biological technician. After a series of tests, Dick was diagnosed with Alzheimer's disease at the age of 85.

Marion and Dick very often travelled to the United States and during their last trip, Marion noticed that Dick was getting confused about directions. They were in a parking lot very familiar to both of them when Dick became confused about exiting the lot. He took a wrong turn and Marion had to direct him. On looking back at that episode, Marion realized that she chose to ignore the warning signs. She was frightened but didn't wanted to admit there was anything wrong.

As time went on, it became evident there was something very wrong. They first attended the True North Clinic for memory testing and Dick's memory loss was noted. Dick was advised to try medication, which he refused.

For some time, Marion let things go and tried to convince herself nothing was too terribly wrong. However, three years ago she finally made an appointment with a geriatric specialist. A driver's test was set up immediately. Dick became very confused taking this test. However, it was three months later before a letter was finally received from the Department of Motor Vehicles asking Dick to surrender his driver's licence. Marion stated that the driver's test had cost $460. Dick was formally diagnosed with Alzheimer's at the age of 85.

Dick had always been the primary earner in the family, travel companion and in charge of the finances. As well, when he retired he bought the groceries and did the banking early on. Marion was her husband's "secretary," as she described it. She organized their trips, community activities and connections with family and friends.

Marion described having a very dominant mother who controlled most of her activities. On reflection Marion felt she had lost confidence and found it difficult to make decisions. As a result, she felt she procrastinated in dealing with Dick's memory loss. She mentioned how kind and gentle Dick was and how he never became violent. However, he did become frustrated when he realized how confused he was.

As Dick's dementia progressed their roles reversed. Marion took over the family's financial role and Dick became more passive. During the three years at home, Dick tried to do small chores around the house but progressively became less and less able to complete any small manual tasks.

Mary

Mary was married to Max who died of Alzheimer's disease late in life. Max developed dementia as a result of the treatment he received for brain cancer. After the dea,th of their spouses, Max, who lived in British Columbia, and Mary, who lived in Nova Scotia, re-connected at a university reunion and struck up a long-distance relationship. During a visit by Max to Nova Scotia, he and Mary decided to marry. Before they were married Max told Mary that he had multiple myeloma — a cancer that starts in plasma cells. At that time, Max was symptom free, but he did require regular treatments. They found the medical support between Nova Scotia and British Columbia to be seamless, so Max's condition did not concern them significantly for a number of years. At a certain point there was some spread of the cancer, and Max had chemotherapy to try to hold that in check.

Mary had not observed significant changes in Max prior to receiving chemo treatments. However, following chemo Max indicated that he would like to write a book. He spent a good deal of time on his writing and when Mary checked his progress he had completed a title and five lines. She thought perhaps he had writer's block but when she read the five lines they did not make sense. For the first time she began to wonder about his cognition.

Shortly after this Mary developed shingles in her eye and she required drops to be administered regularly throughout the day. Max attempted to give her the drops and Mary quickly realized that his vision/perception was not accurate. While she was recuperating Mary had to arrange for someone to come in to do the tasks that Max could not do, including meal preparation and driving.

When she recovered from shingles Mary made it her mission to determine what was happening to Max. After many consultations, a gerontologist they were referred to concluded that Max's brain had been affected by the chemotherapy. From that point on there were obvious signs of both physical and mental deterioration that resulted in a diagnosis of dementia.

Mike

Mike is a 32-year-old geologist living in the HRM area of Nova Scotia while his parents reside in a large city in Ontario. He is an only child.

His father Eric, aged 72, is living with dementia and his mother Irene has been having seizures — likely, her doctor suggests, because she has been the primary caregiver for her husband of forty-two years.

Eric was first diagnosed with dementia two years ago after his doctor sent him for tests due to memory loss and also confusion. "Dad had a lot of other tests — blood and stuff like that — but everything else was fine." Mike flies to Ontario to see his parents once a month because

> I just feel so guilty that I am not there to care for my dad and mom. I am an only child, and the pressure is really heavy for me to go home. I have always been so close to my dad but now he hardly knows me. I used to identify a lot with him and now, as I am considering when to marry my fiancée, I am worried that if we have kids I will get dementia and then pass it on to them.

When his dad first started to have confusion and some memory loss, he asked his wife to never let him go into a home if the time ever came for that to happen, and she agreed that she would keep him at home. Mike said that while he understands why she did this, he wishes now that she "could get him into somewhere where he wouldn't need so much care from her, for her own health's sake."

Mike noted that many of his roles changed as a result of Eric's diagnosis.

> I have to worry more about them now. I am the one who pays the bills when they come in; I do all the banking for them and make arrangements for any medical appointments and I make arrange-ments to get someone in to fix things if needed. Like Mom called to say that the burners weren't working on the stove, so I had to call the electrician and have him replace them. It does cost me more money, but they are my parents. I'm more like the parent now and don't feel like their child anymore. It isn't a great feeling, I can tell you that. Sometimes I wish I was their baby again.

Pam

Pam is an 81-year-old woman who lives in Yarmouth, Nova Scotia. Her husband, Jake, was diagnosed with Alzheimer's disease in "September of last year." He is currently in a nursing home in that county after Pam "had a serious stroke and could no longer care for him." Presently Pam is staying with a daughter in the Annapolis Valley, where she used to live before marrying Jake three years ago. Pam was married before but divorced her husband "due to his drinking. He had been in the military and after he retired, he spent most of his time drinking with his buddies at the Legion. I just didn't want to do it anymore, especially after he wanted to move to Yarmouth where he was originally from." Pam and her first husband did move to Yarmouth, where she "hoped he would stay home more often and keep me company. But that didn't happen. I knew no one there and his family was long gone. So, I just gave up and asked for a divorce." Pam and her first husband had two daughters; one lives in the Annapolis Valley of Nova Scotia, and the other lives in New Brunswick.

After her divorce, Pam met Jake. She had "settled into the town when I was on my own." Jake had never been married and had worked "on the ships as an engineer. He travelled a lot when working and was never interested in settling down with anyone. He enjoyed the single life too much." After Jake retired, he became involved in the local community of Yarmouth. He "played bridge and was really good at it. He was also active in the local Legion, but was never a drinker, and he was a member of a local curling club and the Mariners Centre." Pam met Jake at a curling bonspiel as she also played. She said that they "used to hang out at the [curling] club and after we got to know each other he asked me if I wanted to go out to dinner with him. We just went from there really." After a year, "which we figured was a suitable amount of time at our age, we decided to get married, mainly to make my kids happy. I don't think they liked the idea of me 'living in sin.'"

After they married, Pam and Jake bought a "little house in the town of Yarmouth, which was close to everything we liked to do. We had some friends there because of the curling club and he had friends from his other activities. I also joined a knitting and sewing group."

Pam said the first two years of their marriage was

> *a real adjustment for both of us. He was used to living alone and I was used to living with an alcoholic, so spent most of my time on my own. But we got along well until he started to get confused, disoriented and have memory problems. He kept forgetting and repeating things, as well he kept losing stuff and putting things in strange places. One time I found the iron in the bathroom, or he would put the knives and forks in the cupboard instead of the drawer. One time when he was doing the laundry, he was putting*

the dishes in the machine. I was just coming in from outside so luckily was able to stop him. I wasn't sure at first what was going on. Then after I talked with another gal in the knitting circle, she said that it sounded a bit like what happened with her husband and I should try to get him to a doctor. Her husband was diagnosed with dementia and is now in the same place as Jake.

Pam was able to talk Jake into seeing his doctor. She said that he was

very good at listening to me when I asked him to do things, when he was lucid anyway, so we did go and see Dr. McNeil and he sent us for tests at the local hospital. After the test results were sent to his doctor, he diagnosed Alzheimer's in the early stage.

Pam said that when Jake was diagnosed, she felt as if her life

was really over. We had planned a future together for the rest of our lives and now it looks like I will end up alone anyway. When you get the diagnosis, it is so hard to take in because you know that everything in your life is going to change from then on. You aren't a wife anymore, you are some type of caretaker and it really changes your perspective on how you see yourself.

Pam said that the roles which Jake played in her life were

really equal. We did most of the chores together; I was really clear about that, having been the one in my other marriage to have to do everything. I wasn't going there again that's for sure. Jake was okay with that because he had had to do [it] for himself all of his life. Not that we agreed on everything of course. I didn't like the way he did the dishes; he didn't like the way I did the laundry.

Pam said that when she married Jake their finances were separate. They did "become really good friends. We went on trips together, had many of the same friends, liked the same things like books, movies and music. It was a much better fit than my first marriage."

Because Pam had been married before, where she said that she did

everything — all of the meals, shopping, paying the bills, keeping an eye on the bank accounts, staying in touch with the girls, all of that was up to me — it was a nice change to not have to do everything

*in the relationship. You can't have an equal relationship if one of
you is doing everything.*

Pam is the one who keeps in touch with her daughters and some of
Jake's old friends. She sends out regular emails to their friends and neighbours giving them updates on Jake's health status. She said because of the
COVID-19 pandemic "I have been unable to see him for months, and after
the stroke I had to move in with my daughter because I couldn't use my
left side at first. It is better now but I do get twinges which worry me."
When Pam had her stroke, she was

> *forced to put Jake into a nursing home. I didn't want to do it but
> neither of my girls could be expected to take him in and he couldn't
> live on his own anymore. It was such a dreadful time; I was wor-
> ried about me, worried about him and missing him so much. I did
> get Shirley [her daughter] to buy him an iPad so that he could see
> me sometimes on that FaceTime thing, but he had to have help
> at the home to show him how to set it up and he doesn't really
> understand when he can see me and hear my voice, but I am not
> there. He cries a lot too and that is so hard on me. Half the time he
> doesn't know who I am anyway, so I do it less now than I used to.
> This Alzheimer's is such a dreadful disease and it hurts everyone
> involved. I really hate it.*

Reg

Reg lives in Dartmouth, Nova Scotia. He is 85 years old and he was the
main caregiver of his wife, Nell, who died two years ago in a nursing
home after she had been diagnosed with "vascular dementia and clinical
depression." Reg said,

> *At first I wasn't sure what was going on as she had been diagnosed
> with the depression about two years before the dementia diagnosis.
> I thought her mood swings and memory loss were the result of the
> medications they had her on, but then it was obvious that something
> else was going on. I was told it was difficult to diagnose dementia in
> people with depression, so it was a real hurdle trying to get answers
> from our family doctor and also the ones in the hospital.*

Reg and Nell had been married for forty-seven years. He said,

She is the love of my life. The first time I saw her at a dance at the Legion in Dartmouth, I knew she was the one. I know no one says that nowadays, but that was how it happened for me. I was lucky that she felt the same way, and after a courtship of three years I finally popped the question and she said, "Yes." Her parents were so glad I finally got the courage to ask as they were starting to doubt my intentions I think.

Because Reg assumed that Nell's initial changes of behaviour were related to the medications she was on for clinical depression, he was skeptical of the diagnosis they were given.

They had her on Zoloft, which often gave her headaches and insomnia and she would get so restless not being able to sleep at night and just wandering around not knowing what to do with herself. It was hard to watch, and I just couldn't seem to get her out of it. Of course, it got much worse when Josh [their son] moved away, and she wanted us to move to Australia to be closer to them. But I wanted to stay here where we knew people and where our friends were. I did think when she was at her worst that she would just go to Australia and leave me here. But that never happened.

Other than the above symptoms Nell also experienced

severe memory loss. She was sort of paranoid and was having delusions, mostly about people trying to get at her. She was often getting confused too. Some evenings we would do puzzles together, and she would get really upset when she couldn't concentrate on where the pieces fit. She had a system where she always put the corners on first and sometimes she would be so frustrated when she couldn't find them.

When Nell's symptoms "seemed to get worse," Reg said that he was

devastated because I sort of had a feeling it wasn't just the depression, which was bad enough. I had friends at work whose husbands and wives ended up with dementia and even Alzheimer's, so I had some idea of what was going on. It is so scary to watch someone you love die before they die, before they physically leave the earth.

Sarah

Sarah's mom, Lillian, was a former teacher, a no-nonsense mother and a modest woman. She lived on her own into her eighties until a medical condition required that her daughters help her. The medical condition turned out to be an inoperable mass originating in her uterus and involving other organs by the time that she was seen by a specialist.

At this point her daughters were in their fifties and moving home to care for their mother was not an option. Lillian agreed to move approximately three hours from home to live with her daughter Sarah. Sarah was 58, had married a widower two years before and was commuting an hour daily to teach at a university in Halifax. Sarah's husband had cared for his wife as she died of cancer and Sarah was concerned that caring for her mother might become too great a burden on their marriage. In spite of her reservations, she and her husband moved out of his home and reclaimed Sarah's house, which she had been renting out since her recent marriage. There they set things up to care for Sarah's mom.

Sarah's mother's dementia came from the medication she was given to cope with the growing mass. "It was a catch-22 — we could get rid of the dementia if we ceased using the medication but the uncontrollable pain that resulted left my mother with no quality of life."

Sarah's mother arrived in September and she was "quite sensible" at that point. Sarah continued to commute to work four days a week and, with her husband in the home, most of Lillian's needs could be attended to. As her needs increased they hired a neighbourhood woman to stay with Lillian through the day. She was not trained in care provision, but she had raised a family and could cope with Lillian's growing requirements through the fall. When the caregiver started working with Lillian she was able to play board games. As time progressed she still wanted to play the games, but the rules changed daily until while playing Scrabble none of the words were actually words.

By November Sarah had cancelled her scheduled sabbatical to work in the US and negotiated to take the winter term off to care for her mother. Nighttime care was an issue. Lillian would get out of bed and urinate on the carpet oblivious to the fact that there was any problem with this. She had signs of paranoia and was concerned about a strange man in the house (Sarah's husband).

At Christmas, family photos were taken and they told a story about Sarah's mom's deterioration. She was not in any sense her typical self.

What struck Sarah most was the change in her eyes — they had lost a "knowing" that never returned.

Sarah had inherited her mother's modesty and having to deal with her mother's bodily functions was a stretch for her. "In reality my mother and I reversed roles. Where she had been a loving but 'no-nonsense' mother to me I became her loving but 'no-nonsense' caregiver."

Shirley

Shirley, who is 81, and her husband, Bill, moved to Nova Scotia from New Brunswick twenty years ago. They moved to the Maritimes from the State of Maine in the US after Bill was given a job as an administrator for a small town in New Brunswick. After ten years there he was offered a similar position in Kings County, Nova Scotia, and they moved to a small community overlooking the Bay of Fundy because

> we used to come to Nova Scotia in the summers and when we accidentally drove here, on our way to Margaretsville and getting lost, we fell in love with the area. We asked a real estate agent to look out for a place for us here and after we had rented a place in town for a year he found this cottage, so we moved right in and loved every minute of it.

Bill was diagnosed with Lewy body dementia and died of a heart attack three years later while living in a nursing home.

When Bill retired, they travelled back and forth to the US to visit their children and grandchildren and on one of those visits their daughter Marion, a nurse, asked Shirley if she had noticed that Bill seemed to be going through personality changes.

> One minute he was up, the next he seemed depressed. He often seemed a bit confused too. I said I assumed it was because he was going through missing work and the roles he played there, where he was an important person. I thought he would improve as he got more used to being retired. Because we only saw the children a few times a year when we went there or they came here, she agreed that might explain his behaviour. But she did suggest I keep an eye on him. As time went on I did notice that he seemed to be getting forgetful and he did sometimes seem disoriented and confused. I worked as a counsellor in a nearby town, so I was trained to deal

with different types of behaviour, but it is different when it is your
husband and you are so used to his ways.

As Bill's memory continued to deteriorate and he became depressed,
Shirley talked to her daughter who came to visit and at that time and she

urged him to see a doctor to make sure there were no underlying
health reasons for his symptoms. Marion was always his favourite
"Daddy's little girl," so he agreed to do that. After tests he was ini-
tially diagnosed with Lewy body dementia when he was in his late
sixties, but later in the disease he was diagnosed with Alzheimer's.
Marion and the other children wanted us to go back to the States
then but we were happy here and wanted to remain. I chose to stay
at home to take care of him and did so for more than four years
until I got cancer and had to take him into a hospital because my
doctor told me I couldn't do it anymore. It was the hardest decision
of my life and I still feel guilty that I did that.

Shirley said that as Bill's health deteriorated she faced

many hurdles with him. After I had washed, dressed and fed him I
used to take him outside to sit in his favourite chair in the garden,
so I could make the beds and clean up the dishes. He used to fall
asleep in that chair and one day I went out to check on him and
he was gone. As you know our house overlooks the cliff and even
though there are bushes at the end of the garden, I was worried he
had got through them and fallen the thirty to forty feet over the
edge. I ran across to the neighbours and they helped me look for
him. We found him about half an hour later at the back of their
property [across the street] and he was stuck in the woods; he was
all scratched up. He was very upset and was totally lost. It was the
saddest thing. I was beside myself with worry and guilt and felt
like a bad person for leaving him out there alone. The neighbours
helped me to get him home and after that I called one of the local
men who does construction and had him build me a wooden fence
at the back of the property. Another neighbour worked for a sheet
metal place and he built me a fence around the property as well. It
was expensive but I had to keep him safe.

On another occasion while Shirley was getting gas outside a nearby grocery store, she had left Bill in the car when she went to pay for her purchase. When she returned to the car

> *he was gone. I always locked him in when I did that and I had to take him with me to buy the groceries because I couldn't leave him at home. I found him walking down the road, not too far away. After that, through my contacts in the health community locally I was able to find a young man who was a CCA but had quit working at a nursing home to do online psychology courses at home. I paid him to come to the house when I needed to shop. Bill was not comfortable with women carers so I had to find a man. He worked out very well.*

Shirley spoke about how difficult it was for her to care for Bill at home. She wanted him to be cared for at home but,

> *he would wake up at all hours of the night and wander about. When I would go to the kitchen he would be trying to put the kettle on for a coffee and he would leave it plugged it and then forget what he was doing. One time he was putting flour in the coffee maker so I had to put the kettle, toaster and coffee maker in the cupboards and get those child locks put on the doors. As well, I had a neighbour put a chain on the front and back doors so he couldn't just wander out. All of this made me feel like I was a jailor in his own home and I can't tell you how guilty and ashamed I felt. But I did think I could take care of him better at home than have him in a nursing home.*

Sonia and Andy

Sonia and Andy are a mother and son who care for Sonia's father, Stan (who Andy calls "Grandy"), who has vascular dementia, in their home in Annapolis County. Andy is eleven years old and Sonia is "at the other end of my thirties." Sonia suggested that we interview Andy because "there are many kids in the support group we go to who help their families take care of other people in the family and we need to recognize their needs and their supportive care."

Andy thinks his grandfather is "really old. He's about 66 or maybe even more." Sonia confirms that her father is 66 and he lives with her and Andy. "I don't think anyone recognizes how difficult it is for kids to see someone they love not know who they are anymore. I didn't want him to be frightened so I teach him how to help me and Dad." Andy said that *one Christmas, Grandy's friend Mike gave him and me a baseball hat. His said "Grandy" and mine said "Andy" because that's my name. When Mike went to get the hats made, the guy said that he couldn't fit "Grandad" on the cap, so he put "Grandy" instead. So, we're Grandy and Andy and we think that's so cool.*

Andy, Sonia and Stan live in a small town in the Annapolis Valley. Sonia works as postal clerk. Her husband left her when she decided to take in her father to care for him after he was diagnosed. "Jim was always the jealous type and he didn't even like it when Andy was born and needed more of my time than he was getting. I was just glad when he left because it was too much for me dealing with his stuff, my dad and Andy." Andy was going to school until the pandemic closed the schools in March 2020, but he is hoping to go back to school in September of the same year. He said that he "really misses" his

friends and teachers and last year we had a pet rabbit that we were taking care of. "Hops" we called her. Our teacher Ms. Atkinson took her home, so I want to see her again; she was so cute. I wanted Mom to get me and Grandy a rabbit but she said no as we don't have time to take care of one.

While at home Andy helps his mother by "doing the dishes; I dry them up. I cut up stuff too, like carrots and cauliflower and Mom lets me help with the pancakes on the weekends. They are my favourite and Grandy's too, but he likes his with brown sugar. I like maple syrup and banana." Andy also reads to his grandfather when he gets home from school. While not at school Andy said he reads to his grandfather "every day. His favourite is Harry Potter. Mine too, and I take him outside to play too. He sits in the garden in his chair and I play on the trampo[line] or bouncy castle. Mostly he just falls asleep and I play." Andy also assists his mother with Stan's everyday routine activities such as

after Mom gets Grandy up I get his cereal. His favourite is Cheerios but I like Froot Loops best, but I am not allowed to have them every day. I pour out the milk on our cereal but Grandy is messy and sometimes spills so I have to clean his face with my face cloth. I help with lunch too, and at snack time I put out the nuts and raisins. Grandy doesn't like raisins so he only gets nuts.

Since Stan moved in with Sonia and Andy, Sonia has moved to working part time,

> mostly morning shifts from 9:30 to noon. A neighbour comes in and takes care of Andy and Dad and she brings her two kids in too. Then on other days, when she needs to do errands and stuff I take her two in the afternoons. One of them, Ella, is the same age as Andy and the other one, Emma, is only three. It works out really well for both of us but it is hard on the purse strings only working part time.

When Stan worked, he

> worked for a cement company. He was gone a lot working in New Brunswick and other places in the Maritimes and I know when he retired he missed the work and friends and the travel. Stan's wife died of breast cancer in her late thirties. About the same age I am now, so of course I worry about my own health all the time. I was just a young kid when she died so I hardly remember her. My aunt Edith took care of me when Dad was away. She lived down the street and I always came home when Dad did. I was an only child. Auntie died two years ago, also of cancer. She was like a mother to me and I miss her every day. She was a big help to me when Jim left — buying groceries, cooking meals and taking care of Andy when I was at work. I couldn't have managed without her.

Stan was diagnosed with vascular dementia after he started to have "short-term memory loss as well as difficulty concentrating and remembering how to get to and from locations when driving. He also seemed to get paranoid about things and was getting delusional, imaging people were going to harm him and that sort of thing." After observing these symptoms and expressing her concern, Sonia talked her father into seeing his doctor, who after ordering tests, diagnosed his condition. At first Stan remained living in his own home and managing "fairly well." But then Sonia saw that he was

> losing weight, getting frustrated and anxious and seemed just sort of apathetic about things he really used to enjoy. Even Andy noticed that his grandad seemed distracted so we talked him into coming to live with us. He had sold his house when I got married and he rented a two bedroom apartment in town. So, he gave his notice

and we got help moving his stuff in here. I thought it was only right he should live here; when he sold his house he gave me and Jim the money to pay off the mortgage here, but he wanted his name on the deed too. So, it was always sort of his house too anyway.

Andy remembers when his grandfather started

acting sort of weird. He wasn't acting right and he forgot things. We used to play games and then he would forget the rules and just make stuff up. Mom said not to worry him about it so I just said it was okay. I always used to beat him at Snap and Go Fish and Crazy Eights but then he kept forgetting how to play.

Andy said that he was

very happy when Grandad came to live with us. I knew Mom was sad about him and I used to see her cry sometimes so I was happy when he came to live with us. I love Grandad and it is sad that he is not well, but we love him just as if he was the same as before.

Sonia said that Stan had been a

very loving and supportive father when he was home. He taught me how to fish, although I never caught anything and then he taught Andy too. He made Andy's first train when he was just a little boy and he was always really good with him. He used to go stock car racing with some friends from work. Sometimes when he was older he would take Andy and they were quite a team. Dad was good with the finances and could always fix anything that got broken in the house. I miss that about him now because we never spent a penny on repairs and maintenance; I would just call up Dad and he would show up with his tool box and fix the problem.

Andy said that Grandy was

super. He took me and my best friend Dylan [a neighbour who attends the same school as Andy] for ice cream down at the corner store. He took us to baseball too, and he always came to our games. He does still come sometimes but now but he forgets the rules and gets kind of frustrated.

Andy said that Grandy also used to take him and Dylan

camping some weekends. We would go just the three of us. He showed us how to put up the tent and we would try to catch fish to cook on the fire. We hardly ever did, so then we had to have hamburgers which Grandy brought in the cooler. We also made s'mores and marshmallows. It was so cool and so fun. We could swim sometimes too, but Dylan doesn't like being in the lake. He thinks there are things in there and I know there are 'cos Grandy said so, but I pretend I don't know.

Sonia said that now she plays the role of the "co-sole caregiver, because Andy is such a big help and he seems to like being able to take care of Dad." Sonia organizes all of Stan's doctor's visits; helps him get up, bathed and dressed every day; and helps him to get ready for bed. He is not at the stage where he needs help with going to the toilet and she is grateful for that. He is also able to have a bath, "not often, about once a week and then Andy sits with him and they play with boats in the tub. They are like a couple of kids together really and it is cute to watch them." Sonia pays all of the bills and manages the household finances for the family, as well as shops and cooks all of the meals, with Andy's help as previously mentioned.

Andy has specific chores. He said,

I take out the garbage every two weeks. Mom sorts it but I take it out. I help with getting our food ready. Sometimes I help Grandy do up his zipper 'cos he forgets sometimes after he pees and I don't think he would like that. I help make the beds sometimes and I can even fold my own stuff from the dryer. When I get bigger Mom says I can do more if I want and I do want to do that.

Sophie

Sophie is a 54-year-old East Indian woman living in a coastal community just outside of HRM. She and her husband were the main caregivers for her father-in-law, Floyd, who was diagnosed with dementia in 2006 when he was 79 and who died in a nursing home in 2019.

Sophie told us that

in 2005 at the age of 79 my father-in-law had a stroke. In 2006 he was diagnosed with vascular dementia. I noticed that the 2008 death of his [common-law] wife exacerbated the dementia. A neighbour contacted Adult Protection because my father-in-law told her he was going to jump off the wharf (she did not discuss anything with us). Adult Protection suddenly arrived and acted very quickly.

Sophie and her husband had to find a care facility for her father-in law,

because I worked full time and my father-in-law could not allow his son to care for him. We paid for him to be in the Eastern Shore Memorial Hospital in Sheet Harbour until a bed came available [six months later].

My father-in-law was like a dad to me. We were so close; he was my teacher and guide. He taught me about the political world and introduced me to old country music. We had lived next to one another for years and when he moved to the facility, I felt guilt, anger, resentment [towards the disease] and denial that this was really happening.

Verline

Verline is 62 and she has been married to Frank, who is 69, for thirty-three years. They live in their home in Annapolis County. In his early sixties Frank noticed that he was getting forgetful, and when he saw his physician he was diagnosed with frontal lobe dementia. Verline has been his main caregiver throughout the progression of his disease.

After many years of marriage and a very successful career path for Frank, he and Verline moved to Nova Scotia, where she had grown up. The marriage was not exactly "a fairy tale relationship." Frank had a controlling nature and liked being the centre of attention. He made it clear to Verline that he already had children [from his first marriage] and that would not be part of their married life. At one point Verline left Frank but later returned. Frank stood by Verline while she coped with breast cancer and she was very grateful for that.

As mentioned previously, in his early sixties Frank recognized that he was forgetting things. His father's siblings all had Alzheimer's disease, so he was really concerned. He went to the family doctor, who confirmed his worst fears — he was diagnosed with Alzheimer's disease. He was put on Aricept. Frank became very violent and he was referred to a psychiatrist to determine why this had happened. The psychiatrist took Frank off the medication and ordered CAT scans. After reviewing all the evidence, he said that Frank had frontotemporal dementia. It was suggested that it may have developed as a result of a traumatic brain injury — possibly sports related. Frank had ample opportunity to have suffered a brain injury as he played high level hockey without a helmet and he was around farm equipment in his youth which may also have resulted in a head injury.

As time progressed, Frank had more significant memory issues. He gradually lost his speech and he became less able to decipher what was being said. He would become frustrated and throw things. Frank lost all empathy and personality. He could no longer understand times or dates.

Verline asked,

> So, what is my life like now? I feel like a mother caring for a toddler. I have to ensure his safety, do all the household tasks, look after the finances, drive him where he needs to go and come up with simple activities he can do on his own. He naps in the afternoon and sleeps through the night, so I have that advantage. I also don't feel that I am in danger as Frank is never violent.
>
> Even though I live with a person who looks like a man, my life as a "woman" has ended, and I get sad about that. My brother sometimes asks me, "What's your plan?" I answer, "Survival and it is not going to get any better."

Viki

Viki is 62 and lives in Shelburne County. Two years ago her mother Irene died in hospital at the age of 82 with Alzheimer's disease. Prior to the diagnosis of Alzheimer's, when she was 76, Irene had been treated for clinical depression and she also had bipolar disorder — both possible precursors to dementia — so her diagnosis was expected.

Viki's mother Irene married early and always had mental health issues. Years later when her husband left, Irene's mental health was even more significantly affected. Viki said that her mother was sick for as long as she can remember and that Irene was often "confused and depressed and spent a lot of time in her bed. It was hard to recognize the symptoms of dementia." She did notice that Irene's memory was

> getting very poor and my sisters said that too. I did take some time off work to stay home with Mom and then a neighbour who used to be a nurse said that she would come in and be a caretaker for Mom

two days a week, so I paid her to do that. She too noticed that Mom was getting very forgetful and even more depressed than usual. At first we thought it must be all the meds, but then it was clear that it was something else. So I took her to see the doctor at the clinic here and she ordered some tests, which confirmed, as well as they can, that it was some sort of dementia, probably Alzheimer's. At the time, it was not as shocking as I thought it would be because we sort of expected that Mom would get something else for us to worry about. I work in the health field and I had heard many other people's stories that sounded like Mom's.

Irene was 76 when she was finally diagnosed with Alzheimer's disease. Viki said that in so many ways her mother was

more like a child than a mom. She did the best she could considering her health, but my sister Jo was more like a mother to us as she was the oldest. Mom and Dad were sweethearts in high school, and they got married young. Mom was only 19 when she had Jo. Dad was gone a lot for work so Jo had to do all the household stuff, pay the bills, buy and cook the food, take care of us. That's why I didn't so much mind taking care of Mom at the end. I always felt like I was mothering her for the last two years of her life — dressing her, bathing her, doing her hair, feeding her, taking her to medical appointments, reading to her, watching out for her — you know, all those sorts of things you expect a parent to do.

Discussion: Noticing

What do these stories tell us about "noticing" dementia and the impact on caregivers? As we are introduced to the caregivers' narratives we see that there is no standard path to recognizing that a friend, neighbour or family member is developing dementia. Some of the warning signs of dementia highlighted in the narratives were

- an inability to plan things or follow through on plans;
- difficulty communicating and, in particular, finding words;
- difficulty remembering factors related to the passage of time including the time of day, the day of the week, etc.;
- memory loss;
- apathy and loss of interest in things the individual used to enjoy;

- challenges with complex tasks (including driving); and
- challenges with motor skills.

All of these are classic signs that an individual may be developing dementia. They are also signs that can be easily explained away until they get worse or do not go away with time or changed circumstances; this can cause a delay is assessment. As well, because of the popularly accepted stereotype that older people have "senior moments" or are expected to be forgetful, it is sometimes difficult to accept that their symptoms and behaviours are more than these indications of typical aging.

We also noticed that it was more difficult for family members who did not live with the person displaying these signs to pick up on them or to recognize their potential seriousness. This denial sometimes prompted the person noticing the signs to question their perception or to get frustrated with those who were offering long-distance opinions.

Another reason that caregivers reported in their stories for not picking up on the signs of dementia was the pre-existence of another mental health issue such as depression. Depression is a mood disorder while dementia is a brain disorder, but there are aspects of each that can look similar and as a result one can be mistaken for the other. A recent analysis of longitudinal studies from the *Psychology Today* website titled "Depression and Dementia" (Mani 2021) also shows that depression can contribute to the development of dementia. This is another reason why the careful monitoring of older people living with depression is very important.

A couple of caregivers spoke of a diagnosis coming following a fall. This can occur for three reasons. First, a fall may prompt a more thorough review of the individual's health and signs of dementia may be picked up in that assessment process. Second, dementia may affect the individual's depth perception and this may result in more tentative and unreliable steps. Third, persons with dementia may be more prone to falling because of changes in their gait. The staff of Caring.com have found that people with dementia may exhibit a noticeable change in their walk. They note, "A shuffling walk can also be an early sign of a loss of muscular coordination as the part of the brain governing motor skills (the parietal lobe) is affected. The brain and body don't communicate well. The person has trouble picking up his or her feet to walk and may be unsteady resulting in falls" (Caring.com Staff n.d.).

A Statistics Canada Health Report (Wong, Gilmour and Ramage-Morin

2016) found that caregivers of persons living with dementia are almost equally likely to be spouses or adult children. Spousal caregivers are more likely to be female (58.3 percent); however, male spouses constituted 41.7 percent of caregivers. Among adult children caregivers, 71.5 percent are women. These numbers point out that while caregiving is still predominately a women's role it is important to look at the impact of caregiving on both men and women.

There have been a number of studies that look at the difference between caregiving provided by male partners versus that provided by female partners. A study published in 2019 by Dutch researchers Joukyle Swinkels, Theo van Tillburg, Ellen Verbakel and Marjolein Broese van Groenou explored the concept of caregiving burden in light of the expectation that partner caregiving in old age is likely an extension of women's social role earlier in life, whereas for men it is a new, unfamiliar role.

It became clear in the study that because women seemed to have a greater commitment to the caregiving role, this gave them less time for other activities for which they were also responsible. In addition, they have more secondary stressors than men. Secondary stressors were defined as relationship problems with the person receiving care, financial concerns and concerns around balancing the caregiver role with other responsibilities. The researchers found that the male partner caregivers were less used to providing care than women and therefore experienced the time they spent on caregiving as more burdensome. However, men experienced less stress from the secondary stressors. This type of study is useful in predicting the range of supports that might be helpful while recognizing that stress may be different for male and female partner caregivers (Swinkels, van Tilburg, Verbakel, Broese van Groenou 2019).

Some of the younger caregivers who shared their stories had children and jobs in addition to their role as caregivers, and this positions them in the "sandwich generation" — people, typically in their thirties to fifties who are still responsible for bringing up their own children while also caring for their aging parents. This term is written about in a 2017 report from the Vanier Institute of the Family by Nathan Battams titled *Sharing a Roof: MultiGenerational Homes in Canada (2016 Census Update)* (Battams 2017b). Now, due to higher life expectancies, it was possible for family caregivers to be caring for their elders and their children, and in some cases their partners, in-laws and siblings. The Institute suggested if the analogy of the sandwich was going to be used, it ought to include a "double decker sandwich" and a "hero" as well. On a CBC Halifax Radio broadcast on February 4, 2021, during the *Maritime Noon* program, a phone-in was held with Norah Sphinx, the chief executive of the Vanier Institute of the Family. During the show, several caregivers called in to share the complexity of roles which they were playing, especially during COVID-19. Some were caring not only for family members, but also neighbours and friends. Others were caring for children who they normally did not have custody of — since during COVID-19 the children could not return to the other parent — in addition to caring for adults within the home, some of whom were living with dementia.

In some of the narratives in the "noticing" chapter, caregivers referred to "role reversal." The person who had been cared for or supported by their parent, partner, friend or grandparent is now the caregiver. It is important to recognize that as much as the caregiving may be a reversal of roles, there is a significant difference. Children who are being cared for are generally encouraged to develop increasing levels of independence while persons with dementia are encouraged to maintain existing independence knowing that this gradually wanes as the condition progresses. This progression of loss can have a huge impact on the caregiver.

The diagnosis of dementia as described in the caregivers' narratives often took a long period of time and multiple assessments. This foot-dragging in diagnosing dementia can be stressful and may result in a delay in seeking information, receiving appropriate treatment, making plans, ensuring safety, finding supports and consulting the individual living with dementia about their desires and preferences. In a 2009 study conducted by Pimlott, Persaud, Drummond, Cohen et al. entitled "Family Physicians and Dementia in Canada Part 2. Understanding the Challenges of Dementia Care," physicians were asked why they encountered challenges in diagnosing dementia. According to the physicians' responses, Pimlott et. al (2009: 509) state that the delay was often due to

- substantial uncertainty about making the diagnosis;
- limited access to specialists;
- office visit time being insufficient to undertake cognitive assessment;
- the complexity of diagnosing dementia compared to other chronic conditions;
- the "artificial environment" of the physician's office;

- uncertainty around the management of dementia once the diagnosis is made; and
- differing viewpoints between the individual being assessed and their family members.

There is hope that the introduction of memory clinics throughout Nova Scotia will make assessments for dementia easier to access and the expertise required to offer treatment and support options for the individual and the caregiver(s) will be more readily available (see Chapter 6 for more information).

In some of the caregiver narratives there was a hesitancy to get an assessment for dementia, either by the individual showing signs or the caregiver. This is not surprising because of the stigma attached to dementia. The Alzheimer Society of Canada has an excellent section on stigma related to dementia (Alzheimer Society of Canada n.d.d). They address the causes and manifestations of the stigma including the use of stereotypes and misperceptions, misleading assumptions about dementia, belittling jokes about people with dementia, fear of negative reactions and concerns about stigma by association. As a result of the negative light in which dementia is represented in social media and public perception, individuals and caregivers may avoid accessing an assessment for dementia.

The Dementia Strategy for Canada (*A Dementia Strategy for Canada: Together We Aspire*) acknowledges that the best quality of life for people living with dementia and their caregivers requires timely access to assessments, diagnosis and treatment as well reducing stigma and discrimination around dementia (Government of Canada 2019).

3

Responding

In the next section of questions to caregivers, we discussed their responses to the news of their important one's diagnosis, the impact becoming a full-time caregiver had on their own health and wellness and the effect this had on their self image. Another component of these topics frequently raised by caregivers was their sense of isolation (especially during a pandemic), fear, anxiety, exhaustion and the difficulties associated with taking on new roles, sometimes those held by the person they were caring for.

Amber

As the only child of a single mother, Amber had the sole responsibility for her mom, Joeleen.

> *My role really changed. For so many years I was the kid; suddenly I am the mom, and it was a real challenge. No one teaches us how to parent our parents, and Mom could be right stubborn at times. I had to buy her clothes and she never liked most of my choices — not colourful enough she would say. She loved bright colours. She didn't like some of the stuff I cooked too — too many veggies she would always say. I was trying to make sure she got good food but she liked her chips and stuff like that.*
>
> *I kept Mom at home when she was sick. I did have the VON people come in to help her with daily stuff, like washing herself and that. They did a bit of cleaning and sometimes would heat up the lunch I left for her. I needed to work to bring in money and I did find it a lot of work to take care of Mom, but she deserved it as she had been a single mom to me and now I was the same for her. Mom never changed towards me as she got sicker, not like some of them. She always knew who I was. I got sick a few times because of the*

*stress of taking care of her and working and worrying about what
would happen if I couldn't take care of her anymore. We didn't
have to pay for the VON so that was a good thing, but towards the
end I had to take time off work to just be with Mom every day. I
have great bosses and they were really good to me about all of that.*

Anne

As her brother returned home and Mac's condition declined, Anne
arranged for more household help, adding food preparation and medication management. The caregiver started calling every day with stories
about things that Malcom was doing — giving away money, telling people
his credit card numbers and driving. When Anne confronted him about
his driving, he shot back, "Well, I only drive on Saturdays." Anne arranged
for a driving test and Malcolm failed. She removed the car and her father
became very angry.

Anne knew then that she had to take the next step and move him
out of his house to a place where he would have more care. This began
the "dance of the moves." Malcolm's first move was to a privately owned
assisted living facility. There were a number of his former friends and colleagues there, so it was a great place for Malcolm to continue the social
life he had enjoyed. Anne's brother from Ontario came back to help with
the move. They developed a transition plan where they slowly got his
apartment ready and Mac was comfortable with the move. What Anne
did not know was that all Mac's Scotch whisky from his home moved with
him and was stored in the back of a closet.

His friends observed that while Malcolm had been a great card player,
he was no longer competitive. However, they continued to invite him to
play and Malcolm gave no signs that he realized he had lost that skill.

Mac could not bathe and dress himself, so these services were purchased from the facility. The caregivers started to complain that Mac was
aggressive, and that was nothing that Anne had seen in her lifetime with
her dad. She was really puzzled. One day she discovered by accident the
closet with the Scotch whisky and it was filled with empty bottles. Mac had
been drinking with no monitoring! She removed all the bottles. Things
seemed to improve when the Scotch was gone.

Mac had always loved walking and he would walk in the area around
the facility, always finding his way back. Concern about these walks
coupled with previous aggressive behaviour resulted in the management

contacting Anne saying that her father had to move. Anne noted that at this point she was driving an hour to have a half hour visit with her dad, so she found another private facility in the community where she lived and moved him there. This worked well for a period.

She arrived one day and someone said, "Your dad loves bingo." Anne's immediate response was that her dad had always hated bingo until she realized that he probably enjoyed it now because it involved numbers, which had been his life. Eventually Malcolm's wandering became an issue again; one day he disappeared and the police had to be called. Following this the facility owner suggested that Anne move Malcolm to a long-term care facility. In the meantime, while they waited for Malcolm's assessment and placement, Anne was required to hire someone to be with him twenty-four hours a day. She registered him in an adult day program to keep him active for part of the day, and she found she learned a lot about adult day programs as a result of his participation in this program.

Malcolm was placed in a "horrible facility" more than an hour's drive away from Anne. The deal was that if he stayed there temporarily, he would be assured a bed just forty minutes away when a new facility that was under construction opened. On the day that he was to be moved to the new facility, Anne was given a time to come and pick up her dad. She arrived right on time to find that he was there waiting alone — everyone else had already been moved. Her heart broke for her dad who must have felt totally abandoned. During the short time he stayed at this home Anne noticed that he deteriorated significantly. For example, he arrived perfectly able to look after toileting and left there incontinent.

The next facility was much nicer, but Malcolm stayed only a short time because space became available in a new long-term care facility in the community where Anne lived. In the new facility Anne was stopped the first week Malcolm was there and asked how long he had been on Ativan, which is a drug used to treat anxiety and seizure disorders. She had not realized that he was on Ativan — there had been no discussion about this with her. At Anne's request Malcolm was taken off Ativan and Anne noticed that he became more active and engaged. He participated in recreation activities and was more social. Anne called the previous facility to ask why she was not made aware of the fact that Malcolm was on Ativan and was told by the administrator, "We don't tell the families every little thing we do."

Anne found that the new facility generally had caring staff and she took her dad out every weekend until that became impossible. On weekend drives Malcolm often wanted to see his "home." Anne came to realize that "home" was his childhood home, and she would take him there. They would sit outside and talk about his experiences at home.

When the staff called to say that Anne's father was dying she was caught off guard. His health had been deteriorating, but without communication it was hard for her to determine how far he had slipped. Toward the end of his life the staff made a decision to stop feeding him, but this was not communicated to Anne. One day she was feeding Malcolm and he was opening his mouth and licking his lips when someone came in to ask her to stop and said that he was not to be fed anymore. One staff member said, "Surely this is not a surprise." She found this comment demeaning and unnecessary. Anne spent Malcolm's last evening with him and he died in the night. Anne was glad that he had a private room because they could leave Malcolm in his bed until she got there in the morning.

Betty

Betty is a 76-year-old widow. She is a retired administrative assistant who cared for her widowed mother Deb who developed rapid onset Alzheimer's disease when she was 74 years of age. Betty did not provide the location in which she cared for her mother, who died in a long-term care facility.

Betty was to meet her mother at Deb's apartment and go to a church supper together. As Betty was leaving her home the phone rang. Deb was on the line saying, "I am going crazy! I was supposed to go on a picnic, and I don't want to go!"

Betty immediately rushed to her mother and found her totally confused and panicked. Betty called an ambulance and Deb was taken to the hospital.

As Deb was going through x-rays and various tests, Betty dashed back to her mother's apartment and searched through her cupboards and closets for alcohol or drugs. She found none. As Betty arrived back at the hospital she was told it was suspected that Deb was developing rapid onset Alzheimer's at the age of 74. In this case the diagnosis came in a hurry and Betty was shocked and panicked. The doctors explained to her that this disease displayed two deaths: one mental and one physical. It was explained to Betty that Deb needed sixteen-hour care immediately and Betty realized she couldn't look after her mother. She had a husband, a young son and a full-time job.

Within a few days, Deb was whisked off to long-term care. Betty was told by her other family members that she was in charge of her mother's care and responsible for all the decisions around it.

Betty found herself in the roles her mother had always taken. Deb was a strong-willed woman, trying to meet the needs of all in her family. She was the matriarch and now everyone looked to Betty to take on that role.

Betty felt overwhelmed, lonely and deserted by her family and church community. She was told she was "selfish to put your mother in a nursing home," but no one offered to help her. Betty's immediate family consisted of eight people, all of whom needed Betty's attention. Betty neared exhaustion trying to meet everyone's needs.

During this challenging time, the long-term care facility Deb had been placed in was proving to be totally inadequate. It was poorly staffed, dirty, with poor food and inadequate personal care. Adding to all Betty's other responsibilities, she now had to find a clean and safe place for her mother.

Fortunately, Betty found wonderful care for Deb at a nursing home in Dartmouth. There the staff took great personal care of Deb; the food was nutritious and the staff kept Betty informed about Deb's situation. Betty visited Deb three times a week. Betty remembers the staff calling if the weather was foggy, snowy or not safe for her to drive out to see Deb.

However, all the happy activities which Betty and Deb shared — shopping, church suppers, going to church, drives and so on — were now impossible. All the life-giving fun events ended abruptly, and Betty was left with overwhelming responsibilities, decision-making, anxiety and sadness.

During the third year of Deb's illness the final blow came one afternoon when Betty walked into her mother's room and was immediately screamed at. "What are you doing in my room? Get out! Who are you anyway?" Betty replied in shock, "Mom, I am your daughter!" Deb screamed at her, "No, you are not!" Betty remembers that two staff members heard the conversation and took Betty aside to comfort her and explain that this is how the disease works in some cases.

On looking over the four years of her mother's illness, Betty indicated that she felt her confidence had diminished, and she was still feeling the doubts about how she handled the situation.

Brenda

As time progressed Clifford became more unsteady and after a couple of falls, homecare services were increased. Clifford had a habit of yelling at the workers, particularly when he was confined to bed. Brenda's approach to the homecare staff was simply that this was her father's home and he had mental health issues, so if the workers had difficulty with that maybe this position was not a good fit.

When he first started on full-time care it was recommended that her father go on anti-depressants, as her dad was said to be "combative." As he was never physically aggressive (they were referring to his yelling), Brenda said no; this would change the nature of what her father always was. As a result, he does take medication for sleep, daily aspirin and medication for prostate, but that is all.

At the time of the interview Clifford had been in bed or a wheelchair for six months. Brenda believes that he still understands most of general conversation and has maintained basic social skills although he rarely initiates conversation. At one point Clifford began to ask for cigarettes. Brenda limited his cigarettes to three per day and he managed to get someone else to purchase cigarettes for him. She realized then that while challenged in many ways, he can still communicate when he might benefit from the communication. Another example of this is when other family members visit Clifford and they talk between themselves about things that are happening in the family or community. Brenda will hear snippets of these conversations from Clifford later.

Some days Clifford almost seems to be totally lucid again. One of the home support workers commented to Brenda, "Your father's functioning seems to have reversed. His responses today were accurate and clear." Brenda brought this up with the doctor who visits her father. "Can there actually be improvement in conditions like this?" she asked. "I really don't know," he responded.

Claire

Claire identified herself as a

> dutiful daughter. My father was a hard task master and he expected my brother and me to do well at school. We went to a private school in HRM and then we both went on to university. Other than that, we didn't really have other roles we were expected to fulfill until my mother needed help.

Claire hired a care provider for her mother and found a suitable private nursing home for her. Besides that, no other respite care was needed. While there were financial costs involved in her mother's care, the family was able to afford them "without issue." Claire said that her role as the organizer of her mother's care and later her father's care was

> *challenging at times as I had no knowledge or experience of doing that kind of work — interviewing strangers to take care of a parent, arranging a salary and making sure they were comfortable in the home. So it was rather scary and I did a lot of second guessing myself that I had done it correctly.*

Dale

Dale continued to visit her friend Peggy regularly in long-term care. As time progressed, other people started to notice changes in Peggy, but dementia was never discussed. They would say things like "Peggy is just not herself" or "Peggy doesn't seem to want to discuss politics anymore." But people danced around any discussion of dementia.

> *Peggy was in LTC for just over two years and she went from being able to carry on a conversation to virtually no engagement. I would hold her hand and read her the newspaper. Sometimes I would help her eat too. Her skills were pretty good but if I stayed over the supper hour I usually found some way to help. I felt that I had lived through a cycle with Peggy — she started mentoring me and in the end I would be there for her.*

Deanna

Deanna's grandmother, Riet (Oma), was initially able to stay in her own home.

> *Mom and her brothers paid for a private homecare woman to go in every day and help her with some of her activities, like getting washed, toileting, buying groceries, helping her clean up and that sort of thing. When she wasn't able to stay in her own home anymore, Mom had to get her a placement in the home.*
>
> *There were costs involved in taking care of Oma. Mom and her brothers divided the cost between them and fortunately they could afford it. When they sell Oma's home, which they*

will not do while she is alive, they will be able to recoup the costs of her care.

Deb and Cathy

Both women said that as the dementia became more progressive so did their parents' confusion and forgetfulness. Although, both say that "it comes and goes. Sometimes they know who we are and what's going on; other times it's like we are strangers." Both women said that as the symptoms increased so did their parents' reliance on them, and they both felt "overwhelmed and guilty for not having them come live with us, and scared of them having to go into homes."

Cathy's dad, Ernie, also lives at home and she used to see him daily. As she said,

I used to go over every morning to get him up. Then I helped him wash and get dressed, and then I would make his breakfast. He has one of those emergency bracelet things so he can reach me anywhere, anytime. He used to have the VON but they only had women workers and no Black people. And he hated being taken care of by white women, so I talked to the pastor of our church and she asked in church one day if there were people who could volunteer to help me out. Can you believe thirteen people volunteered, including three high school students? They were all women but he didn't seem to mind that so much. Then two years ago one of the church ladies lost her husband to cancer, and she didn't want to live alone, so she moved in with him. That took a lot of work off my shoulders, but she is 90, so I do need to go over every day to check on them, just for my own peace of mind you know.

Diane

Diane is from a large family who are scattered across the country but are in close contact. She said,

I am the eldest of five siblings, so we did our best to consult with each other about Mom's and Dad's care needs. Three live away and one sister lives just outside town. My sister who lives near would be the primary support during the winter, when my husband and I would go south, and I would take over in the summer. This worked well, but as Dad's dementia progressed I no longer wanted to winter in Arizona, although my husband did, and while this created some friction in our relationship, he did agree to stay in the province. I felt guilty leaving my mother, even though my sister was here and my mother wanted me to go. I felt torn between my husband's need to go away and my need to stay in Nova Scotia to care for my family. When placement for Dad became inevitable, my sister wanted to care for him in her home. She did not fully grasp the twenty-four hour, seven days a week nature of the job, nor was her home set up to provide the necessary care. Eventually we agreed on placement.

Donalda

Donalda had to leave her job in order to care for Grace because, as she said,

Right now, since I stopped working, I am her full-time caregiver. I help get her up in the morning, put her to her bed at night. I pray with her, and if Brandon is home he does too. Sometimes I get Jessie to read to her, but she doesn't always like that because she forgets what the story is about and gets him upset because she thinks the people in the books are people she is supposed to know. So she asks him questions about them, and he keeps telling her they are people in a book.

As well as being full-time caregiver to Grace, Donalda also

keeps the house, feeds everyone, I do all the grocery shopping, wash-ing, ironing, cleaning — everything that needs to be done. The kids and Brandon help when they can, but the young ones have their own lives to live as well. If she has to go for medical check ups, I take her on the bus. I don't drive and that is a real challenge. She don't like the bus and gets really cranky when we have to go on it. When we have extra money, I get a taxi to take us. Luckily, we don't have to go that often for appointments and now we have the von saying that they are going to come in soon to help with her daily washing and hair. That will be a big help because they can do the blood work while they are here. They haven't come yet but are supposed to soon.

Donalda said that she used to be active in the community and her local church, but because she "is too busy now with everything I have to do around the house and take care of Grace, I don't have time for anything else, including sleep."

While Donalda and her family have not yet received support from outside agencies in Grace's area, they have been assessed by the VON and are waiting to hear when a CCA will be able to go to the house to assist with personal care and some other duties. Meanwhile, "some of the ladies from the church do come to visit when I need to go and get my hair cut, or take one of the boys to the dentist, or doctor or something like that. They will come and sit with her while I am gone."

Donalda said that she was told by the assessor who came to talk with her and Grace that there would be no costs involved in the services they provided. She did say, though, that

> we have to buy the adult diapers for her now. She is on a special diet because of the blood pressure and medications, so our food budget has gone up. When you are feeding boys, they eat a lot! She has to have more fruit and vegetables now and they are expensive when not in season. We also have to pay the taxi fares, so it is putting a strain on our budget. Grace and Tyrone never owned their own home so when she moved in with them, she didn't bring a lot of money into the home, just her OAS and GIS and Tyrone's small pension from working on the docks off and on. His health was never really good.

Donalda said that she often feels stressed and overworked with all that she has

> on her plate. I didn't mind taking care of the kids, but I never expected to be doing this too. But I know the Lord puts these things in front of us to see how well we can manage, so I don't like to complain. I do feel exhausted sometimes though when I go to bed, especially with one ear out always listening for her to call me.

When asked if she has learned anything from the experience of taking care of Grace, Donalda said that she

> was blessed to be able to do it. We all love her so much. The woman she is now is not who she really is, or used to be, and she didn't choose to have this sickness. I know if things were reversed and it was me that was sick, she would do whatever she could to help

me. I just wish it wasn't happening. It is especially difficult for the boys, who have to live with this every day. They don't get what they need, I know that, but there are only so many hours in a day. I keep them well fed, washed, they always have clean clothes and good meals, but I know they miss me and their dad and the life we used to have. When they weren't out on a Saturday night, we would get in a pizza and watch some TV or get a video and they really liked that together time.

Donalda said that her faith and that of her family has helped them deal with Grace's Alzheimer's, and she sees it "as God's gift to help us be good to each other in this time, because you never know, it could be you next." She said belonging to the church has given her

a sense of true community with everyone caring about everyone else and a sense of belonging. You know we African Nova Scotians have had a lot of prejudice thrown at us, and our lives have been hard sometimes, but the Lord and the church have always seen us through, and will see us through this too.

Edith

While Edith did have some support from her daughter and family, she said that the changed roles didn't impact her life. "Those things had to be done and so I did them. It's not like you have a choice." Edith also said that most of their friends and neighbours knew about Tom's health, as a few times she had to have the paramedics come to the house when he had fallen and she couldn't get him up. She explained it this way,

I was in the shower and I left him watching something to do with sports on the television. When I got dressed and came into the living room he wasn't there and I thought I had heard a crash. He had tried to get something out of a cupboard in the kitchen and stood on a chair instead of his stool. Anyway, he fell off and I couldn't get him up. I didn't want to ask the neighbours to help because it was early in the morning and I knew Liz was out so I called the paramedics. They were really good with him and got him settled in front of the TV with no problem. Other than bruises on his back and side he was fine, thank goodness.

According to Edith most of their family and friends were very supportive of her and Tom and some would "come by often with meals, muffins and cookies." Edith said that one of the most important things she learned about herself during her husband's illness was "to realize that it wasn't him acting so weird, it was the disease."

Faye

Shortly into their marriage Bob had a stroke. It did not leave permanent damage, but it was the beginning of an increase in Bob's physical and mental decline. Bob had dealt with prostate problems for many years and as they got worse he was catheterized. The VON came in at the beginning and they showed Faye how to manage the catheter care. At this point Faye was 87 years old, and while she was game to try anything she said, "You really needed three hands to change the catheter and the hand I needed from Bob was never there." She felt that her life was being taken over by bodily functions.

Faye, together with Bob's daughter, applied for Bob to be admitted to long-term care. While waiting for a bed to open up Faye had a "heart event," which she realizes at this point was brought on by stress. Because he was on the waitlist for a bed and Faye's health was being affected, Bob's physician was able to get him into a long-term care facility. The facility that had an opening was more than an hour's drive from Faye's home. In the time that he was there (less than six months) Faye drove to see Bob forty-three times! She would take him out for a drive and would get him in and out of the wheelchair on her own. As winter approached, Faye started writing to the Department of Health indicating that she could not continue visiting her husband once winter driving conditions started and, for the health of both of them, she wanted him moved closer to home.

Bob was finally offered a bed in a small room, with a roommate, in a smaller facility. In order to reduce the number of times he would try to get in and out of bed at night they catheterized him. Faye was able to see him daily, and her visits were appreciated by many of the residents and their family members, who knew her by name. She would play the piano, talk with Bob and read him articles and passages from the Bible. Bob was not communicating at this point, but Faye believed that he knew her.

Bob developed a number of infections related to the catheterization.

After discussions between Faye and Bob's family it was determined that he would not continue in his current state and the next infection was not treated. Within two days Bob died at the age of 90.

Hope

Hope is a 61-year-old university professor who lives in Cape Breton with her wife of ten years. While her wife, Jill, has not been diagnosed with dementia, she does have chronic depression and other mental health issues. Depression can be a precursor to dementia and we agreed to interview Hope because she wanted us to realize that her experiences of caring for her wife, in many ways mirrored those of caring for her 80-year-old mother who has dementia and currently lives in Prince Edward Island. Although her mother now lives in Prince Edward Island, she had been staying with Hope and Jill during the first part of the pandemic.

When asked which roles she played in her relationship with Jill, Hope said,

> *We are both fully employed in professional careers; she is my travel companion and partner in all household chores, routines, care of our pets and decision-making processes. When the depression is most severe and she is sick, I take over almost all daily management and significant decision-making. It was the same with Mom when she was staying here.*

As well as caring for her wife — and her mother when she was visiting — Hope, along with Jill, also care for Jill's parents, who live in a close by community. Hope said,

> *I am actually less social than my wife — when she is well, of course. But if we do plan social engagements, I tend to be the one to organize things: tidy the house, buy and make special food, etc. We do spend most major holidays and special events with her family (mine are in other provinces) and share the responsibility for organizing most of those events when family are coming from out of town, as her parents are now aging and in their eighties.*

Hope said that some of the roles in their relationship have changed, especially when Jill is unable to leave her bed, so that "when she is sick, I am left to do all of the management of the house, make the decisions, organize our finances, care for our animals, cook meals and etcetera. And I still work at my own quite demanding job."

Hope said that caring for Jill can be very lonely and exhausting, as it was with her mother.

> *It can be very isolating and lonely. While she does everything she can, when she is very sick, she is fighting to stay alive. Most people don't see how sick she is, so don't realize how her illness impacts her, me, us, our house, our routines, our relationship, everything. And when she is very sick, as she was last year for more than six months, she is also exhausted, so was in bed by 6:30 almost every evening. This meant that I was up on my own for several hours each night and too tired from being and doing everything, including my job from home, to want to find any kind of socializing opportunities. So, I watched a lot of television during that time.*

We have chosen to include Hope's interview to remind ourselves that caregiving of any type, especially full time when necessary, is a challenging time for everyone concerned and Hope was able to identify clear parallels between caring for her mother and caring for Jill.

Jan

Jan, who is living with dementia and managing life on her own, has one son who lives in the United States.

> *Timothy is a screen writer in LA. When I was first unwell he used to come to visit about once every three months and always at Christmas and my birthdays. Before I was too worried to travel and felt outside of my comfort zone, I used to go there. Because of the COVID-19 pandemic he hasn't been able to visit since last Christmas. He was going to come in March, I think it was, but the pandemic put a stop to that.*

Jan now relies on technology to stay connected to her son. "Timothy calls me once a week and we Skype too." Jan's son purchased a voice activated recording device for his mother so that she could speak into it and record her daily activities both to share with him and to assist with her memory issues. She was able to hire a young student at a nearby university who transcribed the recordings into Word files which he would then print for her so she could refer to these to refresh her recent memory.

Jane

Jane is a 66-year-old retired nurse. She was born and raised in New Brunswick but now lives in the HRM region of the province. She lives with her 88-year-old mother Joyce, who, after a stoke, began to experience short-term memory loss at the age of 64; these and other symptoms progressed until she was diagnosed with vascular dementia.

According to Jane, Joyce worked really hard to bounce back after her stroke. She spent time in rehabilitation and the time finally came when a decision had to be made as to where Joyce would go. While she had made great progress, she still had difficulty swallowing and needed a tube down her throat (intubation). As Jane couldn't bear to put her mother in long-term care, she chose to bring her home to her apartment. One of the nurses warned Jane about taking on such care but as Jane said, "I couldn't bear to have her go to long-term care."

During the two years after the stroke, Joyce's short-term memory escaped her at the age of 64. She still recognized people, but she couldn't remember if she had eaten breakfast, if she had brushed her teeth or if she had called Bob (her male friend) or if he had called her. She couldn't remember how to do ordinary chores around the house.

Jane and Joyce were best friends. They shopped together, travelled together and went to movies and concerts together. Jane's time was taken up for the most part by her mother. From time to time Jane's sister would visit, but not often. When Joyce's dementia set in their roles changed. No longer were they good equal friends, but the mother became the child and the daughter became the mother and full-time caregiver.

As well, when Joyce could no longer drive, Jane would have to drive her to see Bob in New Brunswick. Joyce did see Bob one last time just before he died. Joyce's condition went downhill following his death. Jane reported that her mother "talks very often about publishing her short stories written in days gone by." It is a long-term memory that clearly stayed with her.

When Jane tried to have a life of her own, Joyce pouted and was difficult so, as Jane stated, "It is easier to stay at home. I am a twenty-four hour a day caregiver. I am grieving the loss of my mother; the dementia is taking her mind and osteoporosis is attacking her body."

Jane explained:

> *I have no life of my own; it revolves around my mother and I feel that my quality of life is gone. I remember one nurse telling me that I will know when the time is right to put my mom in long-term care. Now it might be that time, but with* COVID-19 *I don't have that option.*

Janet

At this point in Judy's journey with dementia she is living in an apartment on her own but close to her daughter, Janet, who provides daily care and supervision.

In addition to the dementia, Judy has persistent psychogenic déjà vu. She believes that she has experienced everything before. "Her life is literally like the movie *Groundhog Day*." If she watches the news on TV she claims to have seen it before. Similarly, any movie that Janet would like to watch with her, Judy claims that she has already seen. A family member who asked to see Judy's new apartment was told that he had already seen it when he visited the previous week.

Janet has learned strategies to get around this challenge. For example, she will say, "Mom, I really want to watch this movie. I know that you have seen it before but let's just watch it together this time." This gives Judy a reason to watch the movie a second time. While Judy knows that she has memory issues she doesn't seem to be aware of this second condition that distorts her sense of reality.

One thing that Janet struggles with is not being honest with her mother. Honesty and integrity were values her mother taught her, and it seems duplicitous to use approaches that require her to lie. On the other hand, she knows better than to confront her mother's reality. When she does this she can expect her mom to say, "You always have to be right."

Janet attempts to accept her mother's reality, commenting that our society tends to be facts based and that is not necessarily the reality in which her mother functions. She finds that although her mother may get confused about the literal content of a conversation, she is often accurate as to the emotional content and this can affect her. As a result, Janet cannot placate Judy without risking offending her.

Dealing with COVID-19 is particularly challenging for Janet and Judy. Judy wants to exercise her freedom, but Janet is obviously concerned that she follows the protocols to protect her health. She has signs around Judy's home reminding her of things she needs to remember, but she said, "When you leave home and have rules about not touching things, maintaining social distance, masks, hand sanitizer, etc., it gets way too complicated. If there are four steps, Mom is lost at step two."

Janet realizes that she must often be quite strict with her mother for her own protection. To balance this and try to retain the parent–child dynamic, she seeks out ways that her mother can assume the parenting role. "Spending time with my mother has also allowed me to see her playful, goofy side and this has allowed us to connect on a new level. For instance, we have fun dancing together." In addition to household tasks, Janet now looks after getting groceries, making appointments, tracking down information, ensuring that everything with a remote control is still working, attending to finances, taking her mom on short holidays and acting as a conduit for information between her mom and family members. "I would call myself an advocate, planner, entertainment curator, ball dropper, logistical manager, daughter and friend."

Jeff

After his mother was diagnosed with Alzheimer's disease Jeff took on more of the family roles, although he said that her roles didn't really change that much after her diagnosis.

> She has her ups and downs. When she's down I do everything and she seems fine with that. When she's up she wants to help with the dishes, we fight about what to watch on the TV and she wants to play card games but can't remember any of the rules. One of the gals at the clinic where Mom goes for tests told me to encourage her to play card games to help with her memory, even if it was just two or three cards. She also suggested I buy some of the magnetic letters and numbers to put on the fridge to help her remember words.

When asked if he has someone he can count on to help make decisions about his mom's health, Jeff said, "I often talk to my friends about it and a few of them have had a parent, lover or friend in similar circumstances. As well I have friends at the clinic, so I have people I can talk to when I need to."

Jeff jokingly said that he has learned that

I make a pretty good nursemaid. I try to be patient, which is really key when she doesn't know who I am and what I am doing in her house. I am pleased with myself that I am doing so well really. I was scared about whether I could manage, but so far I think I am doing a good job. Sure, it is very tiring and I would like more of a social life, but with the pandemic around I couldn't do that anyway. Mom is good company most of the time and I am happy to be able to keep her at home where she belongs.

Some of the benefits to the many new roles that Jeff now plays in caring for Stella include that

I am a much better cook than I used to be, I am better with our money and paying all the bills, I am much more patient than I used to be and I hug her more than I used to. She used to be sort of embarrassed about it but now she seems to like it. I guess I am more loving toward her now and more thankful to have her still here with me, and be able to take care of her.

John

John has committed to care for Sandy at home, at least for now. As a result, John's life has changed significantly. He said,

Even though we did things separately we used to do lots of things together and now it is all up to me. I'm now doing all the food shopping and cooking. We can't have the cleaner right now because of the pandemic so I have to do that too. I get Sandy up every morning, help her wash and get dressed, then I make her breakfast and make sure she eats it — otherwise she forgets. Then I get her settled in her chair. I make lunch and help her have a rest in the afternoon. I do the dishes and make the suppers too. Because of the clinical trial I am supposed to talk with her every day about what we did that day to help her brain remember things again.

When asked if he ever feels overworked, stressed or burned out by his new roles John said that this happened

all the time. I am just so tired at the end of the day I can hardly stand it. I don't sleep well because I am always listening out for her in case she needs something. It is just too much for one person to do every day and no one prepares you for doing this. My own health isn't great with the arthritis and I worry what will happen if I can't manage anymore.

The roles have really changed in our relationship and they don't tell you that when you are younger. I am having to learn how to be a father, mother, husband and wife to her now. Some days I am not sure which one I am at any given time and who I might be after she's gone.

Kelli

Kelli's mother, Grace, was not doing well in terms of her bipolar disorder, diabetes and dementia. She said she was becoming more concerned about her mother's health and well-being, as Grace was "becoming more and more depressed at the things she couldn't do anymore as well as her dissatisfaction with how the homecare staff supported her." Kelli began to look at having her move to a private care home.

In terms of the roles that Grace played in Kelli's life, she said that her mother

was a really good mom. She made sure I was well taken care of and she was a good wife too. She did have lots of health issues and when she was on the meds for the bipolar disorder she was all over the place. We were a close family when I was growing up. Mom was a good cook; she made some of my clothes and although we weren't really friends the way some kids are with their mothers, I know she loved me a lot, and I loved her. Now when I think of her and the tragedies in her life, I really admire and respect her. I wish I had told her that more often.

Kelli said that her mother

encouraged me at school. She always wanted me to be a nurse because she wanted me to be able to take care of people. She never liked my boyfriends and never liked Brian [Kelli's ex-husband]. She thought he was "beneath me." I married him anyway and she turned out to be right. When Jo [Kelli's daughter] was born he started to be abusive towards me and very jealous of my relationship with the baby, as if it was unnatural or something. After one episode when I feared for my life and that of the baby I left him, called the police and had him charged with assault. He went to jail for a while and when he was in there I divorced him — the best decision I ever made in my life.

As far as her roles, Kelli said that

in so many ways I was always Mom's caretaker and advocate. At school some of the kids teased me about the way Mom was; she could be very quirky when she picked me up, and I always protected her from anyone who made fun of her. While she was in the nursing home and hospital, I made sure that she was well taken care of. I felt more like her caretaker than anything, and in the end like her mean jailor.

I used to be in a bridge group for years. One of the gals at the hospital, another nurse, set up the club a long time ago and talked me into playing with them. I was a good player and wanted to do things to improve my own memory and retain it. Now I worry that I will get Alzheimer's too, so I joined a bridge club here in North Bay.

Kelli said that they "had enough money to pay for Mom's care. I sold her and Dad's house, which was all paid for and well maintained."

As the Alzheimer's progressed, Kelli said that she was

very fortunate to have people at the hospital to talk to, as well as Jo. I felt well supported and even though I was brokenhearted at the time, I did know I had people I could turn to, which isn't to say that my heart didn't hurt and I often felt at a loss, but I was lucky to have people to look out for me. Many are all alone with this situation.

The changing roles which Kelli had to perform to ensure that her mother's health was as well taken care of as could be expected did cause her to

feel exhausted a lot of the time. I knew I could do the caregiving things because I am a trained nurse. I wasn't prepared or ready for the emotional feelings which came up though. Even when you learn all about this disease and its symptoms, nothing prepares you for the experience until it happens to you. I was often stressed; I thought about her every day and her health consumed me sometimes. I didn't sleep well, lost a lot of weight and just generally felt exhausted.

Laura

Laura reported that her husband Jack is a willing worker and as long as he has all the steps laid out he is persistent in completing the job. This means that with support he can still complete many household tasks. However, connecting with people and developing relationships is a problem because the steps are not as clear cut. As a result, he has no friends or social connects outside of those orchestrated by Laura. Laura also feels the effects of a husband who does not understand his role in deepening or even maintaining their relationship.

So, what new roles has Laura assumed because of Jack's "cognitive impairments"? The key roles are those of researcher, planner and social convener. While these were roles in which she took the lead in the past, they are now hers alone. In the last house they renovated she talked Jack through every step of the renovation — she contributed the knowledge; he contributed the well-developed motor memory related to the required skill. At the end of that renovation, she realized that she did not have the energy to continue to talk Jack through all the steps related to maintaining a house and yard, so they sold their home and moved to an apartment in a larger community. She also cannot coach him through the nuances of maintaining a marital relationship, so she has settled for a pleasant and compliant partner. Similarly, she takes the lead in maintaining the connection with family (children and siblings) who live in another province. Jack is content to hear Laura's perspective of how things are with family members and relies on her to issue invitations or plan trips to visit family.

Laura recognizes that Jack's left-hand tremor is only the beginning of the many physical challenges they will live through, but she finds the mental deterioration (that she still believes to be dementia) to be the most fear-inducing.

Ling

Ling's son Thomas tries to visit once a week.

> *He usually brings his fiancée for lunches on Sunday and we order in Chinese food. It is not what we are used to in British Columbia, not as good, but it saves us having to cook. His fiancée, Donna, is not Chinese, and Gao is not happy about that. We are okay with it because there are not a lot of Chinese women doctors in Halifax and Donna is a specialist in the same hospital where he works.*

Ling said that she accepts that caring for her mother-in-law is her

> *duty as a dutiful daughter. It is how we do things at home and all*
> *young women expect to have to do this one day — to take care of*
> *their own parents and those of her husband too. Even today in*
> *China, which is so modern now, these expectations are still there.*
> *I fear this will change soon though. China has many older citizens*
> *and it is going to be important for families to learn to care for them.*
> *Many young women today do not want to do this work. They want*
> *to have jobs with pay and the couples both work so there is no one*
> *at home to care for the babies and the grandparents. In China we*
> *follow the teaching of Confucius which asks us to use filial piety. It*
> *is an ethical concept which says that it is a virtue to respect one's*
> *parents, elders and ancestors.*

Ling said that although they are not religious *per se* they do follow Buddhist teachings and they are "important lessons for life."

Ling noted that there have been "many advances in China when it comes to the use of traditional Chinese herbs in the treatment of Alzheimer's disease and dementias, but Canada is much slower to accept and adopt these remedies."

After this interview we looked up some of the advances in Chinese medicine regarding the treatment of Alzheimer's disease and dementia and indeed there are many such remedies being used in that country. A brief Internet search found articles from CNN (Zaugg 2019), WebMD (Goodman 2019), Bloomberg Business News (2019), World Health (2019), *American Journal of Chinese Medicine and Science of Natural Health* (Fagen 2013).

Loree

Loree reported that her father, Robert, continued to live independently, but while in Florida she developed a plan to ensure his health and well-being.

> *We arrived home and I met with Dad to let him know that it was*
> *time that someone moved in to help him. Given the design of the*
> *house this should not impinge on his space or prevent him from*
> *doing most of what he wanted to do.*
> *I sent my husband to the church where Dad was still preach-*
> *ing, and he came back with a tale about how challenged Dad was*

following the order of service and delivering the message. At our Tuesday night dinner, I told him that he must resign from the church and not leave the responsibility of asking him to leave to his good friends in the congregation. After a longer discussion than I had hoped for he agreed to resign. Now, I thought, on to the car and his driving …

On Sunday of that week, Dad and his leading lady arrived for a visit after lunch. Dad looked like the cat who had swallowed the canary and finally he announced that he and his friend were getting married. I was not impressed … but there are limits to the role of an "enforcer," so eventually I stepped back and became the observer. The bride was aware of his challenges and still wanted to get married, so with the support of both families, they tied the knot.

For a year Dad's house stood empty. I thought that over that time they would see the wisdom of living in a place that required no stair climbing and could accommodate care providers. However, it was easier for Dad's new wife to work in her own kitchen and Dad seemed to have minimal connection to his home. He was happy wherever his wife was. My siblings came to Nova Scotia, and we packed up and sold his home.

Over the next year and a half, the slow decline sped up and some of the sparkle left his eyes. He sometimes packed his bag and left. He was less able to understand what he read and he was disturbed by watching the news on TV. He still appreciated visitors and loved to go out to eat. However, his nighttime activity was not easy on his new wife, and her family, while patient, eventually decided that he was more than their mom could handle. With his house gone the plan of a full-time caregiver was no longer an option. I accompanied his wife to a placement interview. I was to become Dad's visitor.

Marion

In order to have some time to do the tasks outside the home Marion made arrangements to access some respite care. Following an assessment, she was allotted two hours twice a week to do outside activities, and during this time Dick had personal care including a shower. Marion had her respite care increased to two-and-a-half hours twice a week shortly before COVID-19 settled in; however, when the pandemic shutdown occurred,

Marion cancelled all care as she didn't want to risk sickness coming into the house.

The next big decision came as Dick's condition deteriorated and Marion became exhausted and stressed. Her doctor called her and said there was a place for Dick in a local hospice.

Marion got in touch with both her sons and her daughter-in-law who encouraged her to accept the situation and Dick entered the hospice on June 23, 2020. Marion visits him every afternoon. She now knows how exhausted she was, now that she has more free time and the responsibility of Dick's care has been lifted from her.

Marion's sons were concerned that they were not able to readily visit their father but after a period of time they did manage to visit.

Marion remembers being very bossy and impatient with Dick at times. She missed their joint activities and felt very lonely as she saw her partner disappear before her very eyes. She did feel relief that their income situation did not change. She was able to pay all the bills.

Marion noticed that Dick's friends tended to drift away as the dementia took hold. However, her curling friends and bridge club members kept in touch, and Marion mentioned she didn't know what she would have done without her women friends.

Marion became closer to the boys and her daughter-in-law during this time. While it was very difficult during COVID-19, Marion's sons were in constant communication via the telephone. These calls boosted her morale and kept her going during this isolation period.

Marion had much time to reflect on her life and her relationship with her husband and has spent a good deal of time looking at herself, her life and her responses in different circumstances. She thought not only about the circumstances of her husband's dementia but also the impact of her isolation. This resulted in Marion looking at her life from a different perspective. Where once weak and a follower, she sees herself now as strong, more confident, able to make decisions and "go with the flow" more readily. As well, she has developed a broader and deeper respect for all caregivers. She is more confident in her ability to make decisions. This new confidence Marion has gained has not only given her the courage to face the imminent death of her husband but the ability to carry on with her life as a widow.

Mary

Mary contacted her husband Max's four adult children about his condition, and each of them came from different parts of North America to visit him. When Mary could no longer care for Max on her own, two of his children came to help with his care. They were each able to take time off work to provide this help. They moved into Mary's home and took over many of the routine activities including the personal care. Max was relatively easy to handle through the day, but he was up all night and that was wearing on everyone.

Finally, a son-in-law came to help. This helper insisted that Max live in the "real world." If it was Monday and Max said it was Tuesday he was shown the error of his ways. If this approach of focusing on dates, locations and names were woven into the conversations with Max it might have been helpful, but the constant correcting by this caregiver was more than Mary could handle. She confronted him and this became stressful for everyone.

Max began to become more muddled and paranoid particularly around this assertive caregiver.

Mike

Twice a week the von sends in community support workers to help Mike's mother Irene deal with house cleaning and respite for Eric while she goes grocery shopping. They don't do any personal care because Irene knows that Eric would not be comfortable with that. Mike was not always pleased with the care that was offered to his father. He said,

> I don't know why some of them are called "care providers" because when I was there one time the pcw [personal care worker] was very abrupt with Dad and it was like she didn't "care" at all. I didn't want to report her to the head office though as I didn't want it to have a negative impact on the future care they gave him. Especially with me not being there all the time.

Mike said that there were some costs involved in the care of both of his parents. He pays for groceries to be delivered when his mom cannot leave his father alone. As well, he pays for prescriptions not covered by Pharmacare for both parents to be delivered to their home. He has costs involved with his "monthly trips to Toronto and back and I also have to rent a car when I am there. I try to arrange it so that I can make any medical appointments for them while I am there."

Pam

Pam said,

> We [she and her husband, Jake] were both active in the neighbour-hood. We liked to play cards once a week and I was in a knitting group; not so much now as my eyesight is not as good as it once was. He had his fishing of course and before he got sick he had an ATV [all-terrain vehicle] and he and some of the guys would go for drives in the woods nearby.

Pam said that,

> prior to his memory problems we used to get together with some old friends for brunch after church. We weren't religious but some of our friends were and after the service we would get together for a meal. Sometimes when there was a church breakfast or supper we would do those too, but as his memory got worse he started to be embarrassed and anxious about going out in public. He used to say it made him feel awkward, so then it was just him and me.

According to Pam, both her and Tom's roles changed as the Alzheimer's disease progressed.

> I ended up having to do everything he used to. I didn't mind as I know he would have done the same for me. It was a lot of work though and I was always really tired, what with all the extra work and having to take care of him at the same time. I had to get him up, washed and dressed every morning and then give him his breakfast, lunch and supper, help him go to the bathroom, take him for walks and then get him ready for bed at night. I got Liz to come help me get him into the bath once a week and my, that was a big job.

Pam did have respite from her caregiving work when her daughter would come and be with Tom while she went shopping, for medical appointments or to get haircuts and "sometimes have lunch with some of the ladies from the card games group. I really needed those breaks." As well,

Pam was able to find a place for Tom in a local adult day program and once a week she drove him there so that she

> could get some housework done, change the sheets on the beds, do laundry and ironing — all of those things I couldn't do and leave him on his own. I used to drop him off at nine in the morning and collect him in the afternoon at around three, so it gave me a nice break. On occasion I would meet someone for lunch and that was really special.

Pam said that there was a "small cost" for this service but that "it was worth every penny just to give me a break."

Reg

Nell was the "family organizer" in their relationship, according to Reg.

> Even though I had more time off work, she was the one who planned and organized all the family trips when Josh was young. She kept everything together; she did the bookkeeping and kept me on track when it came to paying bills and all of that. She always baked the birthday cakes for me and Josh and got the parties going. When it was her birthday, we took her out for dinner and then came home and ate ice cream cake from DQ because that was her favourite, and guess who was stuck having to eat it up afterwards.

Reg said that he and Nell

> had an equal relationship. We shared most things, and when Josh lived at home he had his chores too. Other than dealing with having the car checked and the tires changed, which was my job, everything else was equal. I cooked two days a week. When Josh was old enough he did one day, mostly nachos, and Nell did the other days — although she bought the food items, which we added to the weekly list.

In terms of other roles in the family and community, Reg said that he

> played soccer with a bunch of the teachers at the school once a week, in my younger days, and Nell loved to swim. She belonged to a local swim team and she went two evenings a week. We were very

outdoorsy and as a family often went for hikes. We went camping and we travelled a fair bit. Less so after we retired; we just didn't seem to have the interest anymore and mostly went to movies or watched DVDs at home.

Nell's roles did change as the dementia progressed so that Reg had to

take on most of the daily chores, as well as take care of her and make sure she was comfortable. I had to do that on the days when the depression was really bad too, so I already had some practice in taking everything on. I guess most people just don't have a clue about how hard it is to live with someone with dementia, with all the forgetting things and the mood swings and the crying and fear. I wouldn't wish it on my worst enemy.

When it was decided "mostly by her GP, that Nell move into a nursing home," Reg said that he felt

relief that I didn't have so much to do every day, but also guilt that I had given up on her. I knew intellectually that I just couldn't do it all anymore, but part of me felt like I was giving up too soon. It's hard to express how really difficult a decision it is to put someone you love in a nursing home, even though you know it may be the best thing for them. I do miss her about the place though, every day of my life.

Reg spoke about a friend, Ted, whose wife is in a nursing home living with dementia, but because of the COVID-19 pandemic has been unable to visit with her for over five months.

She could not figure out how to use the iPad so they could FaceTime, so he gave up on that ... and she had been good with computers at home and work. My friend called the home every day to see how his wife was doing, and it was always the same, that she was "fine." He felt so helpless and useless not being able to see his wife. Now he is able to visit once a week, if he makes an appointment, but only for thirty minutes and he can't give her a hug. He said he sits across from her in the garden outside and they just stare at each other while she tries to remember who he is. Can you imagine how God damned awful that is, to sit across from the person you love and not have them recognize you? It fair breaks my heart and I can feel the tears on my face. I am so pleased that I didn't have to go through that.

Sarah

In September Sarah's mother moved in with her and her new husband. As Sarah reported, "She was quite sensible at that point." Sarah continued to commute to work four days a week and, with her husband in the home, most of Lillian's needs could be attended to.

Through the winter Sarah was able to stay home with Lillian, who started to develop some obsessive behaviours including filing her nails.

Sometimes the nail file would go missing and Mom blamed people for stealing the nail file. Other times there was a gathering of birds in the backyard and Mom was sure they were elephants.

We just treated her as if her perception of the world was the truth; there was no sense in arguing.

Early in the winter Mom was still somewhat mobile and she would try to leave the house on her own. One day she "escaped" in her night dress in a snowstorm. It took two men who were in the house at the time to get her back in the house — that is how much she fought her return to the house. Mom had regular panic attacks and keeping her calm was a constant challenge.

Eventually Mom could not get out of bed and she died at home in the spring.

Shirley

Shirley remembers the day when she took Bill to the emergency department of the regional hospital as

the worse day of my life. Bill was a big man at six foot two inches and I am only five foot two, so it was even hard to get him into the car sometimes. I did get the neighbour across the street to help me and we got him strapped in. Then I had to ask for help at the hospital to get him out. I told the nurse that I couldn't manage him at home anymore and I had a letter from my GP saying that he needed a nursing home placement because I needed to go into the hospital for a breast lumpectomy because of the cancer. I had put him down for a nursing home bed but none were available and he was on a waiting list. I was also on a list for Home Care but they never came or called to say when they could come. They did take him into the hospital and I left without him. I cried all the way home and couldn't sleep for worrying about him and whether I had done the right thing. He was there for five days before an opening came up in a nursing home in Annapolis. I drove there every day, over an hour each way, to see him and help get him settled. By then I was just drained. I felt like a sponge: I would fill up, squeeze out the pain and then start over again every day. He was in that nursing home for about three weeks and then a vacancy came up in Coldbrook and he was able to go there, so that was much closer to home.

Bill was 72 when he went to live in the nursing home.

Sonia and Andy

Sonia is not active in her community since her father, Stan, moved in with them. She used to

be in a sewing group, you know, a bunch of us would get together to do crafts like knit, quilt or sew. I used to make some clothes for myself; nothing too difficult. I enjoyed it. It was a chance to get out of the house and hang out and chat with the other women in the neighbourhood. I don't have any time for that sort of thing now as I am kept pretty busy at home.

Stan's roles didn't change significantly as a result of his dementia. He can no longer drive but

occasionally he can remember how to fix stuff. Like when Andy's bike wheel was broken he could fix that, but it was just a fluke because mostly he forgets how to do stuff like that. It does seem to annoy him and I am sure he gets frustrated, so I just try to calm him down.

In terms of changes to her role Sonia said that she does

a lot of trying to get him settled, trying to reassure him he will be okay and he isn't going into a home, which he sometimes seems to think will happen. I make sure he eats properly and takes his meds and mostly just try to keep him happy. Andy is a sensitive little boy and can often tell before I can when Dad is upset about something.

Sonia does not receive respite care at present, but she said

if things get worse and he gets more forgetful or anxious I am going to see if I can get the VON *or someone like that to come and help out. It is a lot of work for me and although Andy is so good with him, he is just a kid and I don't want him to lose out on his childhood. It hasn't come to that yet and I won't let it.*

When asked if she ever feels overworked, time-stressed or burned out caring for her dad and Andy, Sonia responded,

Oh God, yes. Some days are much better than others; it's more the emotional stuff that's hard to deal with. Sometimes when Dad gets frustrated at something, he cries and that is hard on me especially. Andy too, but he cuddles him and then he's better. I think it's harder on me because he can't tell me what is upsetting him. I worry he thinks about Mom and her death, or what will happen if he gets worse. I don't sleep well in case he gets up in the night and I want Andy to get enough sleep, especially when he goes back to school. Dad is really going to miss him then and I worry he won't understand where he is. Andy wants to play sports again too if they allow it because of COVID-19, *and if that happens he'll be gone more too.*

Sonia said their family doctor is

very good at explaining stuff about Dad's condition and if there is anything I need to know she is always there for me. She does call every couple of weeks to check on him and we see her once a month to see how the meds are going. Of course, we couldn't do that at the beginning of the COVID-19 *[pandemic] but she still used to phone to check in. The women at the post office are good to me too. The supervisor always asks [about] Dad and has told me many times not to worry about taking time off if I need to. I am lucky in that way.*

Sophie

Following Sophie's father-in-law's admission to long-term care she recalls,

> *I played the role of his advocate during his time in the nursing home. I took care of his financial well-being during his stay in the nursing home [payments to home, medication and taxes]. During doctor's visits I ensured he and his son [Sophie's husband] had a voice and explained what the doctor was speaking about. I took my father-in-law to community events and encouraged socialization within the nursing home. I organized his clothing to make things easier for staff and himself. Finally, I ensured birthdays and Christmas were celebrated. It was a bit of a balancing act as I wanted to be present for my father-in-law, but I always respected my husband's direction as I did not want to overstep.*

Sophie's father-in-law became more dependent on staff, his confusion and anxiety increased and he would see bugs crawling around.

> *As there were no bugs, my husband pretended to be the exterminator and remove the false bugs. We found that more and more we needed to validate his reality.*
>
> *Sometimes staff had to do more checks and an alert bracelet was on his shoe as needed. Whenever he wore his hat inside it meant he was trying to leave, and the staff would know to watch him carefully. He would remember his son but not me and vice versa, and ask about family members who had died, especially his mother and my parents. While he seemed to be seeking companionship, he chose not to socialize as much and was sleeping all the time.*
>
> *I think for the staff it was quicker for them to conduct his ADL [activities of daily living]. For example, they would use the electric shaver and get him dressed. I would organize his clothes [t-shirts, pants and long sleeved shirts on hangers] to simplify things for staff and possibly allow him to dress himself. Staff shortage was an issue; they did not have the time to allow him to conduct his own care.*
>
> *As the dementia progressed my role in supporting my father-in-law in long-term care did not change as much as my husband's did. He was in more contact with the staff and frequently visited. I always maintained my once-a-week visit but would stop by and*

speak to staff more frequently. During palliative care we were both more present.

I felt stressed by the advocacy role within the nursing home and their lack of age-appropriate recreational activities. Every family meeting we had to educate [the staff] about his directives to donate his body to science.

Sophie spoke of the need to make some personal changes because of the caregiving. For example, "We stayed closer to home and took separate vacations. I would travel [visit her family in Ontario] and we would not tell my father-in-law I was going [because he would worry]. My husband would go on hunting and fishing trips. Again we would not tell my father-in-law because he would worry."

Verline

Frank would become frustrated and occasionally he would throw things. Frank lost all empathy and personality. He could no longer understand time or dates. Verline knew that she needed help and reached out to the von, continuing care and an adult day program.

From the von Verline and Frank were able to access a couple of hours of housekeeping each week. Frank liked having new faces in the house and while he could speak, he repeatedly shared the story of his marvelous life with the home support workers. Verline noted that some of his stories were accurate and some were not.

As time progressed Frank had more significant memory issues. He gradually lost his speech and he became less able to decipher what was being said. In spite of this, Frank loved going to the adult day program which was offered at the local college. He had the capacity to concentrate for long periods of time on things he could do, like puzzles, so he enjoyed opportunities to engage in new activities at the centre. Unfortunately, covid-19 resulted in the adult day program being closed.

Viki

One of the ways that Vicki sought to manage her response to her mother's diagnosis was to see a counselling psychologist. She said,

The year before Mom died, I saw a therapist to help me manage it all. She suggested that I keep a journal of all the things I did on a

daily basis for Mom and how I felt in myself. Here is a page from that journal that I thought you might like to see as an example of a day in the life of a dementia caregiver:

6:00 a.m. get up, go to Mom's room [my house is a three-bedroom bungalow, all on one level], wake her up, have a chat with her to see how she is — sometimes she thinks I am someone else — but I never know who, so I just feel invisible to her a lot of the time. I change her Depends [adult briefs] which she hates, so she fights me, hits at me and yells. Then I give her a bed wash — just her face and hands and her privates. At night I give her a bigger wash. Then I help her get dressed, which is difficult as she used to be a great dresser. Mom was a gorgeous woman when she was young, but now she is too thin and weak. I brush her hair and help her with her walker to go into the kitchen. I had to have child locks put on all the kitchen cabinets and drawers so Mom doesn't get into stuff. I have to remember when I go to bed at night to put the kettle and toaster in the cupboard.

One night I forgot and Mom went to the kitchen at 1:00 a.m. to make scrambled eggs for our breakfast. She tried to break into the cupboard to get the frying pan out. She banged the kettle on the cupboard, it broke and she was sitting on the floor sobbing her heart out because she wanted to surprise me with scrambled eggs. My heart just broke for her. I sit her down in her usual chair and sometimes, if she is "up" I let her help me make breakfast. Usually oatmeal, toast and coffee for me, tea for her. I cut up her food so she can swallow and help her to eat. After that I wash her face and hands and take her into the living room where she sits in her chair and watches TV or falls asleep while I clean up.

We don't talk much — she repeats herself all the time and it drives me crazy. She normally falls asleep so I can read or just sit and watch her and worry about how I am going to manage every day. I make lunch, repeat the morning's activities and then change her diaper again and clean her up — the same at supper time. We watch TV until about 10:00 p.m. when I get her ready for bed again. She often wakes up at all hours of the night. I had to have locks put on all the doors so she can't go outside. It is like she can escape at any moment if I don't watch her constantly.

I think about my childhood with Mom. When Mom was up

[manic] she was a real laugh; she played games with us, took us on walks, took us to play in the park, we went to movies and shows. Then she was a great, but exhausting, mom. When she was down [depressive] she stayed in bed and hardly said a word to us.

Student Voices

In the fall of 2020 Jeanette was asked to facilitate a class at a university in Halifax where the students were discussing death and dying. Jeanette's focus was on the impact on caring for someone with dementia (which was recognized as a life-limiting diagnosis). Her questions to the students were, "If an important one in your life was diagnosed with a form of dementia and you were to be the primary caregiver, how would your life need to change to accommodate this work? What do you imagine your everyday life would look like? What do you think would be involved?"

The following summarizes the students' responses to these questions:

- All agreed that many aspects of their lives would change. Many said that they would quit their jobs or school or, if possible, reduce their working hours. Those who had children still at home recognized that this would be very challenging.
- Most recognized that this work would be emotionally draining. They said they would feel anxious, frightened of the future, exhausted and would have to decide how to find time for the person they were caring for who would take priority, as well as time for themselves and their relationships. People with young children saw this as almost insurmountable.
- Some said that they would spend their time becoming more educated on the topic and try to find out what services were available to assist them and their important one.
- Some said that they would feel frustrated with their situation, that they would need patience and they might question their faith. They also recognized that they might experience guilt and resentment at having to change their lives to accommodate this work.
- Some said that if their important ones lived in another province, they might have to move from Nova Scotia.
- Some recognized that there might be difficult decisions to make with siblings and other family members regarding levels of care and where it should take place and who in the family was available to

provide it, both emotionally and financially.

- Some suggested that they would have to be aware of, and support within reason, the religious/spiritual beliefs of the person they are caring for when they don't hold those beliefs or values.
- Most recognized that they would have to change the physical environment of their own home, or that of their important ones, so that the latter could not wander or get out of the house alone, or cause themselves and others harm.
- Many recognized that they would experience anticipatory grief and loss as the person they loved changed as the condition deteriorated, and perhaps question their relationship to them.

In a follow-up discussion with these students in their regularly scheduled online course, some spoke about their personal experiences with family members who had been diagnosed with dementia and spoke about their "shock and dismay" at hearing this news and wondering how it might affect their own schooling and employment if required to assist in providing care, especially due to the pandemic. Some spoke about observing their parents exhaustion, grief and worry at caring for their parents with dementia and were concerned at what might happen if they had to become caregivers of their parents. Some were working part time while attending classes, while others were parents of young children, also working part time and taking online courses. If they were called upon to provide care, they would be an example of the triple decker sandwich generation.

Discussion: Responding

What do these stories tell us about how the caregivers responded to the diagnosis of dementia and the impact it has had on their lives?

Timeline of Support

Once there was a diagnosis of dementia the stories followed a fairly standard pattern — the first response was generally to determine how the individual with dementia could be supported to live as independently as possible, with the first choice being to support them in staying in their own home. If that was not possible, and the individual with dementia was single, some caregivers opted to have the individual live in their (the caregiver's) home. At a certain point, most caregivers sought help with respite care. This may have involved someone coming into the home or taking the individual out to an adult day program. As time progressed, many caregivers reported that the demands of providing care became too challenging, and they made plans for the person living with dementia to be placed in a long-term care facility. In most cases this involved the person moving to a government-subsidized facility where the charge for care was based on the individual's income. In some instances, caregivers chose to place the person with dementia in a privately run facility. In order to be admitted to a long-term care facility some caregivers shared that they had to have the individual admitted to the hospital first. Hospital admission was usually the result of some kind of crises, but it did have the advantage of speeding up the placement process. Due to the pandemic it was difficult to find a long-term care bed as some facilities were not allowed to take new patients. In some cases going into a hospital was not an option due to the COVID-19 pandemic.

Impact on Caregivers

The caregivers we spoke with were generally spouses or adult children and accepted their new role willingly. While it was not something they had planned for, it was a role they took on without question. Unfortunately, while providing care for children is accompanied by many training and mentoring opportunities, the same is not necessarily true in later-life caregiving.

Unlike other diseases, like cancer or diabetes for instance, dementia affects cognitive capacity and challenges the individual's mental functioning. Caregivers shared that as the condition progressed, activities of daily living (ADLs) like dressing, eating, going to the bathroom or bathing became almost impossible for the individual to accomplish without help. People caring for a person living with dementia are typically left with the responsibility of providing supervision and/or care all day long. As the caregivers noted in their stories, this is further complicated by the need to adapt to the individual's personality and behavioural changes as well as communication problems. It is not surprising that caregivers reported feeling "stressed," "overwhelmed," "exhausted," full of "self-doubt" and "brokenhearted." As one caregiver noted, even the placement of his wife in a long-term care facility did not eliminate the stress, because as much as he felt "relief," he also felt "guilt."

A 2018 article written by Oluwaseyi Rachel Jokogbola, Christopher Solomon and Shanika L. Wilson, and published in *Advances in Clinical and Translational Research, Volume 2,* entitled "Family as Caregiver: Understanding Dementia and Family Relationship," suggests that family caregivers could benefit from a "proper training process and adequate information on dementia and its progression in order to better adapt to the position of a caregiver. Family caregivers need to be recognized as partners in care and caring for the dementia could have adverse effect on their health" (Jokogbala, Solomon, and Wilson 2018: 1).

Commitment to Caregiving

There is a myth that Canadians tend to institutionalize their family members who need extra support. Statistics show this presents a false picture of caregiving in Canada. The Vanier Institute of the Family produces fact sheets on various aspects of family life in Canada. They report (based on data from Statistics Canada) that

> in 2018, approximately one in four Canadians aged 15 and older (7.8 million people) provided care to a family member or friend with a long-term health condition, a physical or mental disability, or problems related to aging. More than half said that they cared primarily for older generations (56%, or approximately 4.4 million total), such as parents, parents-in-law, grandparents and great-grandparents. (Vanier Institute of the Family 2020)

People who chose to provide care to family and friends did so for a variety of reasons. In some cases they spoke of the support they offered as one of the values of their family or culture. A Chinese Canadian caregiver said, "In China we follow the teaching of Confucius which asks us to use filial piety. It is an ethical concept which says that it is a virtue to respect one's parents, elders and ancestors." We saw this reflected in different words when one woman said that she provided care to her mother because she was the "dutiful daughter."

Some caregivers expressed that they were grateful to be able to support parents or partners in their old age. Adult children referenced being supported by their parents as a child and recognized this as an opportunity to reciprocate. An example of this is found in the following quote: "I was blessed to be able to do it; we all love her so much ... I know if things were reversed and it was me that was sick, she would do whatever she could to help me." Partners made similar comments: "I didn't mind as I know he would have done the same for me."

Some of the caregivers who shared their stories with us identified aspects of their caregiving experience as being positive and satisfying. The feeling of being needed and useful in the caregiver role was a comment we saw reflected in a number of stories. Some respondents commented on specific skills they had developed like cooking, managing the household budget and decision-making. As a son caring for his mother stated, "I make a pretty good nursemaid. I try to be patient which is really key when she doesn't know who I am and what I am doing in her house. I am pleased with myself that I am doing so well really."

Finding the Right Programs and Services

When one is faced with navigating the possible options of how best to support a person living with dementia, caregivers have recommended the following three helpful resources:

1. Nova Scotia 211 — Collects information on services and programs offered by government and non-profit organizations throughout the province and provides this information at no charge to callers. It has information on a huge variety of support options and it provides individual personalized help. While this service provides information on a full range of services, "in 2020, just under 49 percent of the 43,000 calls that 211 received were related to support for a senior" (Myette 2021).
2. Alzheimer Society of Nova Scotia — This organization is invaluable in supporting people who are caring for persons living with dementia. A program designed specifically for those caring for someone who is newly diagnosed with dementia is the First Link program. This program connects people who are newly diagnosed to local healthcare providers. People living with dementia can receive information about diagnosis, day-to-day living and positive approaches to care. The program also provides individual support and counselling and links people with the disease to other Alzheimer Society programs and services (Alzheimer Society of Canada 2016).
3. Caregivers Nova Scotia — This organization provides programs, services and strong advocacy for family and friends who are caregivers in Nova Scotia. It operates support groups for caregivers throughout the province and compiles a handbook of resources for those providing care (Caregivers Nova Scotia 2018).

Respite Care

Four options for respite care were highlighted in the caregivers' stories:

1. Seek help from family and/or friends — for instance, in Donalda's story we hear how friends helped out by providing respite care. "Some of the ladies from the church do come to visit and when I need to go and get my hair cut, or take one of the boys to the dentist, or doctor or something like that, they will come and sit with her while I am gone."

2. Receive respite services through the provincial Home Care program — Verline was able to access very limited services through Home Care but it provided a break for both her and Frank. "Frank loves having new faces in the house and he repeatedly shares with the home support workers the story of his marvelous life." Verline notes that "some of his stories are accurate and some are not."

3. Hire an individual who works independently or hire through an agency and pay for the service using your own funds or funds available through another source — Brenda reported that she hires the workers who care for her father, Clifford, with funds provided by VAC. Because she does the hiring it means that Brenda is in control of what happens in her father's home. Clifford had a habit of yelling at the workers, particularly when he was confined to bed. Brenda's approach was simply that this was her father's home and he had mental health issues so if the workers had difficulty with that she would suggest that "maybe this position is not a good fit."

4. Enroll the person with dementia in an adult day program — Edith's story illustrates the value of this service. Edith was able to find a place for Tom in a local adult day care program and once a week she drove him there so that she

> could get some housework done, change the sheets on the beds, do a laundry and ironing — all of those things I couldn't do and leave him on his own. I used to drop him off at nine in the morning and collect him in the afternoon at around three, so it gave me a nice break. On occasion I would meet someone for lunch and that was really special.
>
> Edith said that there was a "small cost" for this service but that "it was worth every penny just to give me a break."

Nova Scotia Caregiver Benefit

A number of caregivers we interviewed mentioned that they valued the Caregiver Benefit, a fund available through Continuing Care Nova Scotia that recognizes the important role of caregivers in their efforts to assist family members and friends. The program is intended for caregivers of low-income adults who have a high level of disability or impairment, as determined by a Home Care assessment.

In order to qualify for this monthly payment, the caregiver must be providing twenty or more hours of assistance with ADLs per week to be a qualified care recipient. In addition, the caregiving relationship with the qualified care recipient must be ongoing. That is, it must be regular and expected to extend beyond ninety days (Province of Nova Scotia n.d.b). More information on this benefit is provided in Chapter 6.

SMILE Framework

An article published on the Canadian Family Physicians website written by Frank Molnar and Christopher C. Frank in April of 2018 and titled "Support of Caregivers of Persons with Dementia" discusses how physicians can support those caring for persons living with dementia. The authors recommend using a framework developed by a caregiver who analyzed and documented how she best engaged with her mother who had dementia. Not surprisingly the framework addresses many of the elements of support we heard in the caregiver stories we collected:

- Stages of life — Just as our parents accept us at every stage of our life as we grow up (baby, toddler, teen, etc.), accept the person with dementia at every stage of their illness. It is better to enjoy and love them as they are now than to get stuck on how they used to be.
- Moments — Whenever possible, caregivers should look for and try to create precious moments. The caregiver who created the framework tries to create or enjoy "a nice moment" three times a day and view any additional moments as a bonus. This can give her a sense of success during trying times.
- Interconnect — Although friends might fall away and family might not always understand, it is important to never isolate oneself. Caregivers should try to turn to neighbours, support groups, information sessions, community services and others whenever needed. The caregiver is not just the caregiver but is also a care coordinator,

connecting and inviting others to participate in the patient's care.

- Laugh out loud — A smile and a laugh can help with responsive behaviour and can be contagious. Finding things that make the person with dementia laugh can help with difficult situations and is good for everyone!
- Experiment — What works one day might not work the next; the caregiver will need to experiment. Experiments should not feel like failure. If something does not work it can still stimulate creativity and collaboration, especially as the person's illness progresses.

In an article from the *Australian Journal of Dementia Care,* author Teagan Bewick of Edith Cowan University (2016) suggests that nurses too can assist caregivers of persons with dementia. She suggests that nurses encourage exercise, socialization, mental stimulation, meaningful activity and to help the person with dementia maintain as much independence as is safe and possible to do. She also said,

> Family can also be hampered by overwhelming feelings of grief for the impending loss, and in later stages, a sense of relief knowing that the journey is coming to an end. A nurse equipped with knowledge and specialised dementia education is capable of providing crucial aid and reassurance to the family throughout all stages of the dementia journey. Nurses can prepare families with educational material relating to respite services and community support services that are available within the community (Hunter 2016). Through holistic assessment and therapeutic communication, the nurse can recognise and address caregiver role strain and coping mechanisms by encouraging regular reflection and maintenance of personal welfare (Hunter, 2016). Finally, the lack of awareness surrounding dementia treatment provision tests the resilience of the family unit as it increases their financial and legal vulnerability. (Bewick 2016)

4

Assistance and Support

In our next set of questions, we talked with caregivers about their sources of assistance and support as they embarked on their shared journey of caring for loved ones with dementia. While some had family nearby, others did not. For those whose important ones had been diagnosed recently, the impact of the pandemic greatly reduced their ability to access services that might have been available previously. In this block of questions, we asked caregivers if they had learned anything about themselves as a result of their experiences; as well we asked if there were perceived benefits of taking on new roles. We also asked if their faith played a role in their experiences, and while most replied that they were not religious or had a denominational faith, some did respond to this question.

Amber

Amber was surprised at how little support she got when her mom died.

> *Other than the people at work who have been so good to me, I don't feel like anyone offered me support or anything. Some of the gals who took care of Mom through the VON did send a card after she died, but no one ever checked on me to see how I was doing or anything. It's like when the patient dies that's the end of their job or something, but they really should check on who's left now and then. We was never religious so we didn't get any help from the church. A lot of the older people who live on the Hill do attend regularly and they get help, but we never did.*

Anne

Anne said, "Every day I was responsible for my father. I felt time-stressed and burdened. I felt that I was the only one who loved him in the way that he needed at that time in his life." This was compounded by the fact that neither of Anne's brothers came to see their dad in the last two years of his life. She said that she communicated with them about every change in care and she had to argue with them constantly to justify her decisions, especially when it involved the expenditure of money. As Malcolm was dying, a nurse said to Anne, "The family members that live farthest away have the most guilt when someone dies." Anne mused that,

It has taken me years to overcome the rifts in my relationship with my brothers. I would ask for help and get no response and eventually I felt that I had lost both my parents and my older brothers. I think things are better now because I have finally forgiven them for not being the way I wanted them to be when I was caring for Dad.

The caregiving role had a huge impact on me — caring for my father became my social life. I had older children who were very active and required attention and support and in addition I had demanding full-time work. I was a single woman who could not think about a new relationship because my available time was consumed with my father. In the eight years between my mom's death and my dad's death my only relationship was a long distance one where I could control the time it took.

Brenda

Brenda reported that almost every day is challenging but every day is also a privilege. She said that if at all possible, members of her family and the African Nova Scotian community in general attempt to care for family members on their own. If Clifford were not able to access support, she believes she would have left the work she loves to care for him. Brenda said, "It is part of our culture to take in everyone and by extension we want to keep family members at home and support them the best we can. I think you will find that a small percentage of African Nova Scotian seniors are admitted to long-term care."

She recognized that her family is "blessed that Dad is a veteran." She indicated that the ability to access services through VAC has made a huge difference to his life and to hers.

Her faith is "everything" to her. Brenda said, "I know who is caring for me and that allows me to care for others." Her coping strategies are "stepping back and refocusing." This involves "asking myself 'What do I need, and how can I make that happen?'" She also takes on "passion projects" that allow her to focus on something else that brings her joy.

Claire

While there were financial costs involved in her mother's care, Claire's family was able to afford them "without issue."

Claire said that their immediate community was aware of her mother's condition, and some were "sympathetic and remembered her fondly for all of her community work. When Mother went into the nursing home, many people were in touch with Father, and he still led a very active social life and did so after her death. He died two years after her due to a heart attack."

When asked if she had learned anything about herself as a result of her mother's disease, Claire said that she found the experience of organizing care for her mother to be

> very difficult and time consuming. I don't know how other people can manage to care for their parents or others at home. It isn't something I could ever have done and I suppose I am lucky that we could afford to hire people to do that. I have lived alone all my life and am happy with my choices. I am confident that I will have enough assets to pay for care should I need it later in my life.

Other than experiencing guilt at having to place her mother in both a care home and then a hospital, Claire said that she felt

> okay about myself in terms of the decisions I was forced to make. I do occasionally feel resentful towards my father for putting me in that place, but he's gone now so I can't tell him any of that and I doubt he would have discussed it with me even if he was still alive.

Dale

Dale reported being "shocked that the family was encouraged not to come to visit while she [her friend Peggy] adjusted to her new home in long-term care. This," Dale noted, "just encourages people to assume that care providers fill all the roles, but they are not friends and family."

Dale found that people didn't know how to respond to the changes in Peggy. "I finally started telling people who were visiting her to expect less from her and bring more to the conversation. I encouraged them to change their expectations but continue to visit; however, I did notice that her visitors waned as the dementia progressed."

Deanna

Deanna noted,

> *Oma was very active in the church; she helped with the flowers and the cleaning, she put out the hymn books and made some of the squares and stuff for after services. At holiday times like Easter and Christmas she made cakes and helped with the teas and things like that. In the summer months, the church put on community breakfasts and suppers and she was one of the helpers and cooks at those. As she got more and more sick, she really missed these times and used to cry when she couldn't do them anymore. The church women especially still visit with her at the nursing home and they help out when they can. It has been really difficult because of the pandemic as none of us could visit with her and even though Mom and Dad bought her an iPad so we could Skype with her, she didn't seem to understand why we weren't there in person or sometimes even who we are.*

In reflecting on the support and assistance from others, Deanna said,

> *My uncles are really upset about their mom's illness. She was always so strong and loving to them. Some of her church friends are a bit worried about their own health. You know, it's like when you hear that someone has cancer and then everyone you talk to has a story about someone they know who has it too. It's like that with Alzheimer's. We have heard about many of the people in the church who have it. It makes you wonder if it runs in families too.*

One of the strategies that has helped her family to navigate the experiences of her grandmother's dementia, Deanna explained, was maintaining open lines of communication.

> *As a family we talk a lot about what is happening with Oma. Even though Mom is reluctant to talk about the future, my dad does talk to her about it, and as a family we share our feelings. I think that lets us all know we are on the same page as to how to care for Oma.*

Deb and Cathy

Both women received care for their parents; in Deb's case through the VON and in Cathy's through the local church. There were no financial costs involved in the care, but they said that there were costs involved in buying their parents aids to assist them live in their own homes.

In Cathy's case she bought an emergency bracelet for her dad to wear and she pays a monthly amount for that. As well, she bought him an iPad so that he could play solitaire and other games during the COVID-19 lockdown. She taught him how to use email too, so he could keep in touch "when he remembered how" with some of his friends.

Deb also bought her mom an iPad so that she could play card games online. Both women said that they had to purchase "Depends, because they forgot to go to the bathroom and the other caregivers were always having to wipe their privates, which they hated." In Deb's case the volunteers who came to the house to care for her dad and his new "house mate" were able to assist with house cleaning, laundry, cooking and such.

In Cathy's case she hired a cleaner to go into the house once every two weeks to do the chores which the homecare workers could not. As well, she made arrangements for a food delivery service to bring hot meals to her mother twice a week, "mostly for her suppers."

Deb and Cathy said that they had good friends to support them, as well as Deb's sisters and they "feel very lucky to have people in our lives who are there for us when we need them. We also have friends who have other family members with dementia, so we support them too." Both agreed that they had "good doctors, who [we] trust." Cathy said that the pastor of her father's church is very supportive and visits her dad as often as she can. As well, she calls Cathy after every visit to let her know how her dad is doing, in her opinion.

Both women said that their neighbours and those of their parents knew about the dementia and were supportive and "always asking if there is something they can do to help." Deb said that her sisters all felt "a sense of guilt" that they are not closer to their mother, but they all telephone on a regular basis and Skype with their mom when she is able to "figure out how to use the computer."

"It has been very hard to change roles from being a child to being a sort of parent," both women agreed, "especially as it is not supposed to be this way. Your mom and dad are supposed to always be the parent, aren't they? It is sort of lonely somehow, because if you are not the kid anymore, who are you?" Deb asked.

We talk about all of this stuff a lot; we feel sad, lonely, guilty, even resentful at times as so much of our lives now is worrying about them, going to see them, waiting for them to get worse, then wondering what we will do about that, then guilty for feeling this way.

"I don't wish this on anyone," said Cathy.

Diane

Diane remembered,

While Mom was alive she received four hours of respite care weekly for which she paid a small fee through Home Care Nova Scotia. She also attended Alzheimer's support group meetings periodically, and Dad attended the adult day program at the local healthcare clinic for a short period of time. Even though Mom and Dad were new to the community, they met people through their church and neighbourhood. People were aware of their health problems and offered support.

When Mom and Dad were home together we interacted daily from April to November [four times a week in person, daily telephone conversations]. From December to March my sister filled this role.

This experience changed how I feel about myself: worry that I could have been more patient with my mother, concern about developing dementia, a sense of satisfaction that I was able to provide care to both my parents in their dying, that they both died comfortably with their families present. I worry about being a burden to my children if I get the disease. It was difficult providing personal care to my dad — he kept repeating himself and that could be frustrating. He woke up all hours of the night and sleep could be hard to come by.

Donalda

Donalda said that she used to be active in work, the community and her local church, but because she "is too busy now with everything I have to do around the house and take care of Grace, I don't have time for anything else, including sleep."

When asked how the experience of being a caregiver for Grace has changed how she feels about herself, Donalda remarked that

> *I knew I was a strong woman, but I never got to see how strong until this. It does make you realize that you can be a nurse, cook, cleaner, friend, daughter-in-law, wife, mother and all those other things all at the same time. I am not saying it isn't hard, but so far, I can do it all. Whether that will change as her health does, and as I get older, I don't know. Right now, I am proud of myself though. I do miss friends from work and that other life, but this is what the Lord wants me to do right now so I am doing the best I can.*

Edith

While Edith did have some support from her daughter and family as well as the Adult Day Centre, she said that she still felt

> *overworked, stressed, anxious and tired most of the time. I had cared for Dave [her first husband] at home before he died, so it wasn't that I didn't know how to do it, but I am older now and it was just too much some days. That was why in the end I had to put him in the nursing home. It was no easy decision I can tell you.*

Edith said that one of the most important things she learned about herself during Tom's illness was

> *to realize it wasn't him acting so weird — it was the disease. So when I would get frustrated, or angry, or even resentful, I had to remind myself of that. Of course, then I would feel guilty that I had those feelings. It's all a bit of a roller coaster really. I also learned that dementia can happen to any of us, so we all need to do what we can to keep our memory fresh. I did try playing bridge because people said it helped with memory, but it didn't help me.*

Edith also said that the experience of caring for Tom and her first husband taught her that

> *I am basically a very strong woman and am good at taking care of other people. I wasn't planning to be a widow yet again and thought*

with Tom that he would outlive me. We used to joke that he would put me in a rocking chair with my knitting and put the CBC on for me to listen to, and then I could just pass away in that chair when I was ready. Even though I am happy now living with Liz and Bob, I do miss Tom every day. He had a way of making me laugh and it hurts to remember the good times we had before his memory went. I am just glad that I am not alone.

Faye

Money was not a stumbling block to accessing services so Faye reached out to the VON for support — they could offer four hours of respite per week, so she started with that. As time progressed Bob was up more at night and so she contracted with a private service to get nighttime care.

When they were not available, she hired someone recommended by a physician. On the night that the recommended caregiver came, Bob slept through the night and the caregiver read in the living room all night. The bill for that service was $400! Faye decided that another solution needed to be found but that solution did not appear, and she started to feel stressed by the responsibility and lack of sleep.

Hope

When asked if she had learned anything about herself as a result of caring for both her wife and her mother, Hope replied,

I originally wrote no to answer this question. Then I went back and erased it, because there have been two benefits. One, we/I have learned to pare back a lot of things that I, in particular, used to think were really important and now I don't. For instance, formerly I would not leave the house to go to a shop without first getting a shower, doing my hair, putting on makeup and nice clothes. Sometimes, now, I brush my teeth and hair and go, because I just need to go get groceries or a prescription. It's not that I don't enjoy getting dressed up, more that I no longer see it as being absolutely necessary to look a certain way before I can go out in public. I've actually become much more relaxed in my attitude toward a lot of things, such as hiring people to do chores and errands, and have found life is just easier because of that. The other major — probably the best — thing to come out of her illness, has been that we talk constantly about absolutely everything — we have to, so that I know how she really is doing, and we can plan accordingly. When we were first together, we each tended to respond to things for the other one — she would say yes to going somewhere she didn't really care to go because she thought I wanted to go (as one example). Now, we sit down and check in honestly with one another before making commitments or decisions. I also have learned to distinguish between what is about me and what is not. Early on if I said something like "Could you empty the dishwasher please?" and then she didn't do it, I took it personally. (Clearly, the things I want are not important.) And I would get angry, empty it myself, crash and bang around, etcetera. I've learned that it isn't that she is unwilling to do it — she has either forgotten (and memory issues are a huge part of her illness) or she intended to but a wave of exhaustion buried her. It was never about me.

Jan

Jan used to belong to a bridge club, but because her memory started to deteriorate, she now plays "'Honeymoon Bridge,' which is just for two players instead of four." She gets together once a week in her unit in the facility with another woman named Connie and she said that "she helps me with my memory problems too. I can hardly remember the cards in my hands anymore, but she is very patient with me."

Jan noted that,

as a result of the dementia, all of my roles have changed and the pandemic has made a big difference too because I can't really get together with anyone. I hope that changes soon as even though I have a few friends here, I don't really have a lot in common with many of them. I do find that some of my old friends are sort of worried to visit me. Not just because of the virus, because we can meet outside, but because they think I will be so different, which I am mostly not, yet. Others seem worried that they will upset me if they ask questions about my health and some seem to think what I have is contagious. People just don't know enough about Alzheimer's.

I have told my son that if and when the disease progresses, which I am told it well may, and if I don't know who or where I am anymore, that I want to apply for MAID *[Medical Assistance in Dying].*

I also told him that if I get a very serious form of COVID *that I don't want to be on a respirator or intubated. I told him, "Just let me go."*

Jane

While Jane was caring for her mother, Joyce, she attended stroke outreach groups and had some help with the provision of personal care from time to time. Very little respite was available, although a social worker did visit occasionally and attempted to help Jane, as well as Joyce. Jane also still had to attend to the tube in Joyce's throat. She couldn't swallow for quite some time. During the first months of Joyce's stroke, occupational therapists, psychologists and recreational therapists came on the scene to attempt to help not only Joyce but Jane as well, as they tried to deal with both the effects of the stroke and vascular dementia. A bed pole was attached to Joyce's bed to enable her to maneuver herself out and the couple had to pay $500 for this.

Jane has one sister who was able to visit now and then, but not very often so Jane was on her own with the care. Jane said that during her mother's illness she "had no life of my own. It revolved around my mother."

When asked what she had learned about herself from the experience of caring for her mother, Jane said, "I have been reflecting on how I want the rest of my life to go. I know I cannot go on like this. I am stressed, exhausted and there is no joy in my life." Jane knows she needs more help in caring for her mom and is planning to be more assertive in getting help for Joyce's personal care and help with the housework. She also plans to ask her sister to care for Joyce for a weekend so she can visit friends at their cottage. Jane also reflected on family history. She remembered that when her mother looked after her grandmother, her mother "changed. I am changing. I am existing. I am losing myself."

Janet

Janet recalls,

> *While trying to balance supporting my mom and holding down a job, I came to the realization that I have a job and it is caregiving. I cut back on many other things in order to give this role more attention. I have to say I was shocked that in all my conversations with the Alzheimer's Society and Caregivers Nova Scotia that no one told me about the Caregiver Benefit.*

Having Mom sit in on the interview to be assessed for this benefit was difficult. One of the questions was "How many hours a week do you help your mom?" I thought of all the things I do while I am with her and then the things I do for her when I may not be in her home and came up with a number. She disputed that number and I felt awkward. How can I encourage her independence and then discuss with someone right in front of her how dependent she is? They need to re-consider this assessment process for persons with dementia.

Being a caregiver is lonely. I sometimes get overwhelmed. I have learned to ask for help but I have also learned to not necessarily expect to get help. There is a lot of social pressure and people offer their suggestions about what I should be doing. I have learned that I can only do the best I am able and that has to be enough.

Jeff

When asked if faith played a part in their lives, he said that "faith has never played a role in my family and we were not churchgoers. I can see how it might be helpful to some, but not me."

John

John said he and Sandy do not receive respite care even though they have asked for it. "Because of the pandemic some CCAs (community care assistants) are choosing not to work, so there is a big shortage of them. We can afford to pay privately and are on a waiting list. But any services like that are not available." Once a week John "goes fishing with other guys near here and the wives come over to be with Sandy. She sometimes remembers some of them and seems to enjoy those visits. Because she forgets her words she doesn't say too much but they fill in for her."

John said that while the people at the facility where the clinical trials Sandy is involved in take place are

helpful when we are there, they can't come home with us and help me there where I really need it. Neighbours help when they can by sitting with Sandy when I go to buy food and other essentials, but they couldn't come during the pandemic, so I had to leave her by herself which really scared me.

John suggested that

some [people] are scared to come to the house now because they don't want to see [Sandy] like that. COVID-19 *has made everything so much harder because we can't have my children to visit, or neighbours and friends, and Sandy doesn't like to talk on the phone. We do have an iPad and I talk with my kids on Zoom every now and then, but she doesn't get how that works and it just confuses her and makes her frustrated.*

Kelli

When asked if her faith played a role in her experience as a caregiver for her mother, Kelli replied that "we were not religious or spiritual in any formal way. In fact at the nursing home they were always trying to get Mom to attend the weekly church services on the ground floor and she hated that. I didn't think it was proper or appropriate either."

Kelli said that the experience of caring for her mother helped her

feel good about myself. I am proud of what I could accomplish. There's no point in engaging in guilt — I have done my share of that. When I moved here to Ontario and the dust had settled, I did go to a therapist to work through my grief and that helped so much. I realize that not everyone could do that, and I am lucky that I still have a health plan through work.

Loree

Loree said that when

my father went into the first facility that became available, not the facility of our choice, he was put in a wheelchair. His gait was unsteady, and we had always worked to accommodate that, but this was not the family's risk anymore, it was the institution's risk, and they decided that he would not be left to walk on his own. I was asked to sign a form allowing for him to be restrained. This meant that he would be tied into the chair. The first three weeks that he was in long-term care I was called three times to let me know that he had "escaped" from his chair — once using scissors, once a knife and the third time they were not sure how he had escaped. The scissors and knife made the possibility of a fall seem rather mundane! I was becoming a cynic.

My father dressed professionally for seventy plus years. When I arrived to visit him at the LTC facility he was often wearing clothing that he would never have worn. I assumed that he was just dressed in whatever was available and when someone died their clothes were shared among the remaining residents. One day I arrived, and he was wearing a cowboy shirt. I laughed because we lived in Calgary for six years and he would not even wear a cowboy shirt to the Stampede. The care team did not know my father.

One of the CCAs told me what a joker my dad was. My dad was a great storyteller, and he was gentle and kind. He was not a joker. He was a poet, an author and a conversationalist. The care team did not know my father.

My father greeted people as they arrived for their meals in the dining hall and he thanked them for coming as they left. One day as we pulled up to the LTC home after a drive he said, "There's my church." He was still providing pastoral care, but no one noticed. The care team did not know my father.

I wondered whether it was important that people know who my dad was or was it sufficient that they make up stories about who he is today. And did this bother him, or was it only bothering me?

Marion

Marion's faith is a deep part of her ability to live one day at a time. She has a broad experience with organized religion. She has worshipped in the Anglican, Baptist and United church traditions. She and Dick were both members of the Presbyterian Church at the time of his diagnosis. She finds great strength in prayer, her mission group and phone calls from her church friends.

Marion spoke about her coping skills. She allowed herself to cry. She spoke about this in great length.

I had to let myself cry. To get all the hurt, frustration, pain and anxiety out in the open. I don't know what would have happened to me if I tried to keep it all inside. By letting it out I was able to make the necessary decisions that had to be made. I would make a decision, have a good cry and carry on.

Talking helped me a great deal. My friends in the Mission Group would call regularly. Respect helped as well. I could go to my bridge club regularly at least until isolation came into effect.

I have discovered more empathy as the days go on. I noticed that Dick would get upset if I was upset. I learned to be calmer and gentler. I was very lucky that Dick was for the most part gentle. I didn't have to cope with anger. This whole experience has led me to self-reflect and look at what advice I could give to other caregivers just embarking on their own journey.

Mary

As Max's dementia and physical well-being diminished, he was cared for at home by Mary and then by Mary and two of his children spelling each other off. After a confrontation with a family member whose approach to care was in conflict with the other family members, a physician interceded and had Max admitted to hospital, where he eventually died.

Mike

Some people like Mike's parents are hesitant to reach out for help. As Mike said,

Although my parents live in a small neighbourhood and are close to the people next door, in general my dad is a very private person and wouldn't want people to know that he is ill. Likewise, Mom tends not to ask for help from neighbours or friends because they think what happens in the home should stay there.

Some friends of long standing do help out. Irene used to play bridge before her husband's health became worse, and sometimes, to give her a break, one of the members of that group will sit with Eric while she goes "to get a hair cut, shop for something for herself, or meet another one of the Bridge group for a coffee, just to get out of the house, you know."

Pam

After her husband, Jake's, diagnosis of Alzheimer's disease in September of 2019, Pam decided to take care of him at home for as long as she was able because she felt that "I owed it to him to take care of him, even though we hadn't been together for long. I wanted him to be safe and comfortable at home for as long as possible." Because they had both "been careful" about money, they did not experience financial worries concerning his care.

The community where the couple lived was aware of Jake's diagnosis and his status in the nursing home he had to be sent to when Pam's own health deteriorated. She said that overall the community had been

> very supportive of both of us. After I had a stroke, and when the nursing home allowed only one person at a time into the home due to the COVID-19 pandemic, Jake's friends made plans so that one of them could visit just to check on him; then they would call or email me to let me know how he was doing.

Pam could not think of any benefits to her new roles as caretaker of Jake, other than

> being able to pull it together when I needed to. I still have a lot of guilt that I wasn't able to keep him at home. I wonder if I could have done something different to avoid the stroke so that we could still be together in our home. There's no point in "what ifs" though, is there? It is what it is, and I have to make the best of what I have now.

Reg

When Reg was caring for his wife, Nell, at home, he said that he did not receive respite care and when the time came for her to be placed in a nursing home there was no public facility bed available, so he had to place Nell in a private facility, for which he paid $3,500 a month. He said that he and Nell's pensions were able to cover most of the costs of the nursing home, but that it is "expensive and I worried, hoping I will have enough to cover all of her costs and mine too if I end up needing to go into a long-term care home, which with Josh [their son] in Oz [Australia] may well have to happen."

When Reg was asked if he has learned anything about himself through the experiences of caring for Nell, he replied,

> The trouble with caregiving is that no one cares for you, so you don't have time for yourself ever and the person who would have taken care of you can't do it and doesn't know she can't anymore. It is such a lonely feeling. I learned a lot of new skills from caring for Nell, like how to be a better cook, how to be more compassionate and how

to be more patient. This isn't to say that I would recommend it to anyone, just to say that you have to step up when the time comes and to try to do it well.

Other than the above, Reg said that caring for his wife in this role made him feel

good about myself, to know I could be there for her when she most needed me. I had a sense of accomplishment sometimes when I went to bed at night, even though mostly I was exhausted. We always had a loving, strong relationship and strange as it may sound these experiences somehow made all that even stronger. I love her so much and miss her terribly now that she isn't here. I miss her telling me she loves me. You know, I know somewhere in there she does, but we used to say it every day before we went to sleep, and I wish I could hear it again.

Neither Reg nor Nell were religious, and he said that the only faith he had was "in myself and what I could do for the best."

Sarah

Sarah was able to maintain her relatively new marriage, hold on to her position at the university and care for her mother by receiving respite from her sister. Every weekend through the fall and early winter her sister from Saint John came for two days to care for her mom, and this breather allowed Sarah to stay in touch with the world and get the sleep she needed to carry on.

Sarah also tried to look for any aspect of "lightness" to get through the caregiving role. She credits opportunities to laugh, visits from friends and the temporary escape from caregiving responsibilities helped her to maintain balance in her life.

Shirley

Shirley said that she and her husband, Bill, for whom she was caring, were not active in community events because she noted that

Bill wasn't a very social person, and when he got sick it was very isolating for me to be with him "24/7." There are various community events going on here, like the monthly breakfasts, potluck suppers,

card games and that sort of thing. But he was very much a home-
body so we didn't do any of those activities. When he was well he
was happy working in the garden, reading local history books and
watching sports on television. We used to go for drives — not far,
but around the shore or into town sometimes. Then we would stop
for lunch and it gave him a break. Before he was sick I was able
to go out to work and also to socialize with some friends. I really
missed doing that when I had to stay home to take care of him. It
was as if my world had shrunk to those four walls. It takes a lot of
resilience for us carers to just keep going day after day, but it does
take a toll physically, emotionally and psychologically.

Shirley said that many of their friends and neighbours knew about
Bill's health and most

were helpful and useful, like picking up the odd thing when I needed
it. But some were also very judgmental about me keeping him at
home and caring for him by myself. They just didn't understand why
I wanted, no, needed to do that. I tried to get them to understand
but I don't think some of them ever did.

Although Shirley did receive respite care for Bill when she went grocery
shopping and for other appointments, she did apply for homecare services
from the VON or a private caregiving agency even though "I knew that
most of them were going to be women and I knew he wouldn't want that.
He was a very private person and although he liked women, he wasn't as
comfortable around them as he was with men." Shirley was able to find a
"trained," competent and caring male to help her with Bill and she paid
him with the help of her children. Even though she and Bill had private
health insurance through their places of work, neither provided in-home
private care. Shirley said, "I knew the care I had arranged was good but
I felt guilty every time I left him with John."

Shirley said she learned a lot of things about herself living with someone
with Alzheimer's disease, including

how to keep things simple for him; not to overwhelm him with
talking and assuming he knew what was going on; how to have
patience with him, when inside I wanted to scream and yell and
cry. I learned how to deal with my guilt over putting him in the
hospital and then resenting him because I had to do that. I also

came to terms with my anger at the system too, for not finding a cure for this wretched disease. I learned how set we were in our ways and how our relationship was sort of stuck in our stereotypical roles and how much I depended on him. For so many years our roles were husband and wife; now they were like parent and child and it is very difficult to parent your spouse, believe me. Because of the Alzheimer's disease and the medications he was on, we were no longer intimate and sometimes he was very aggressive and behaved inappropriately in terms of trying to grab or fondle me or say nasty sexual things. I know it wasn't him but the disease. He was not a talkative person and didn't like to discuss death or dying, so we didn't make what they now call end-of-life plans. Had we, I might have been more aware of what he would have wanted when the disease progressed. I assured the children that I would let them know my wishes and I have.

Sonia and Andy

Sonia shared that her income had changed as a result of her only being able to now work part time, but she said she is

happy to be able to do that for Dad and we have enough to live on what with his pension and some savings. Of course, having to change my life to accommodate Dad has changed everything, but he was a good dad to me and he deserves to have as good a life as I can help him with now. He is only a young man still, but some days it is like he is ancient with all his issues. I feel so sorry for him; I am sure this is not how he saw his life turning out.

Sonia, Stan and Andy live in a

relatively small and close knit community where there are no secrets, especially with people knowing me from the post office. Most people are really kind about Dad. He's not the only one around here with dementia or Alzheimer's, so a lot of customers in the post office tell me about their family and friends and the struggles they are having.

In terms of learning about herself as a result of her father's health, Sonia said that

I have learned so much about myself throughout Dad's illness — like

I am able to do it all is the biggest thing. It wasn't anything I had planned for; I thought I would keep working until I retired, Andy would grow up, go to university or something, Dad would be fine and go about his business and all would be great. Of course, I still want Andy to go to university, get a good job and be happy. I am not the sort of person to complain about life, but I wasn't ready for this, yet it isn't all bad. We are mostly okay. Dad is happy to live with us. Andy is still able to be a kid and he loves helping out. I wouldn't say that there are any perceptible benefits to my new roles, but I am proud of myself to be able to do it all. So that's a benefit I suppose. As well, I have a caring and sensitive little boy who is learning how to take care of people. That's a huge benefit. Maybe he'll be a doctor someday.

Sonia said that the dementia experience has changed how she feels about herself. Andy said the same thing. Sonia said that she feels "I am more tolerant of him now and more used to expecting him to not always know what's going on. I think I have learned to be a better daughter and even mom." Andy said that he feels "good about being able to help Mom and Grandy. It's sort of special 'cos I can do things that my friends can't, like help make stuff for breakfast and the snacks."

Sophie

Sophie noted that when her father-in-law was in the hospital,

only a few people visited. Most of his cousins and neighbours chose to distance themselves from him and us. We had a "date book" in his room. We asked staff and visitors to sign in and write about their visit. That is how we knew about his day, visitors and behaviour. My prayers have given me the strength and guidance I needed.

Verline

Verline could not say enough about the Continuing Supportive Care Grant. The additional money in the household allows Verline have someone care for Frank three or four days a week so that she can maintain her job and attend to her own needs. This program, she reported, is what has "kept her in the game."

One of the challenges that Verline faces is that Frank lost their retirement income before she took over the finances. As a result, money would be an issue if Frank were institutionalized. The partner who resides in the community gets only a portion of the resident's pension and Verline said that this would not leave her enough to maintain the home. Frank is also in that in-between phase where he needs constant care but does not yet need to be institutionalized, so the funding for respite care meets the needs of this couple.

One of Frank's children would be happy for his father and stepmother to live in his home in Alberta, but this is not an option. The other two children have very little to do with their father. Verline can count on Frank's siblings to help. One sister calls daily to check on Frank and cares for him for a week every year giving Verline a week to herself. Verline has used this time to take a vacation south and the siblings have said that they would also pay for her vacation should money become an issue.

"I also have some friends I turn to for support and who I know care about me. It is really important to maintain your own support network because this is a tough condition and people can turn their backs on people with dementia."

Viki

Viki said that she joined a hiking group some years ago, and while her mother lived with her she had one of her sisters come for two weeks every year "so I could get a break and get away. There is a group of us who go for hikes all across the country. I needed to be out of the house and away; otherwise I am sure I would not have been able to cope." Viki said that as supportive of her as her two sisters were, they "couldn't believe how hard it was to care for Mom and her constant demands and needs, so when I got back they really appreciated what a horrible job it can be and what a toll it takes on a person. It is the hardest job you'll ever have to take on."

Discussion: Assistance and Support

The information in this chapter overlaps with some of the responses in the previous chapter as some caregivers responded to the diagnosis by seeking caregiving options immediately (as reflected in Chapter 3) while others delayed the quest to find support until later when the dementia had progressed to a point where they found they needed help. So, what assistance was needed and where did caregivers access it?

Support from Family and Friends

It became obvious from the narratives we gathered that persons with dementia spend considerable time in the community being cared for by family members after the diagnosis. Clearly family caregivers delay, and sometimes prevent, institutionalization. This comes at a relatively small cost to the healthcare system but has a large impact on the lives of the caregivers.

The most significant change mentioned in the stories we collected was the social isolation felt by the caregivers. They missed time they used to spend with friends and family, and many mentioned that they had to give up leisure time pursuits and sometimes employment to provide the required care.

Shirley captured this well in her observation that "when I had to stay home to take care of him, it was as if my world had shrunk to those four walls. It takes a lot of resilience for us carers to just keep going day after day, but it does take a toll physically, emotionally and psychologically."

The support that caregivers reported receiving from family and friends varied depending on prior relationships and the personalities and the unique circumstances of the person living with dementia and their caregiver(s). For this reason, it is hard to generalize; however, we did hear that caregivers who could rely on family to provide respite were extremely grateful for this contribution. Some caregivers suggested that family members who provided respite care also developed greater empathy for the role being filled by the caregiver.

At times the non-involvement or conflict with family members became a sources of stress that compounded the challenge of being the primary caregiver. Anne stated,

> It has taken me years to overcome the rifts in my relationship with my brothers. I would ask for help and get no response and eventually I felt that I had lost both my parents and my older brothers. I think things are better now because I have finally forgiven them for not being the way I wanted them to be when I was caring for Dad.

When family members were not able to provide instrumental care (respite care, help with transportation or household tasks), caregivers reported appreciating emotional support from family and friends.

Small Gestures of Support from Neighbours

Shirley said that many of their friends and neighbours knew about Bill's health and most "were helpful and useful, like picking up the odd thing when I needed it."

While some caregivers reported joining support groups, more commented on accessing informal support from others in the same situation. When we asked Jeff if he had someone to talk with and support him while he cares for his mother Stella, he said that he "often talks to his friends about it and a few of them have had a parent or lover or friend in similar circumstances, as well as friends at the clinic, so I have people I can talk to when I need to."

Deb and Cathy also reported accessing help this way, indicating that it can also be reciprocal. "We also have friends who have other family members with dementia, so we support them too."

Support from the Community

The caregivers shared that some of the factors that allowed them to keep filling their role of caregiver were stores with delivery services, physicians who explained things clearly and checked in regularly and employers who cared about their role as caregiver and were willing to make allowances when that role took priority at times. A couple of caregivers also spoke positively about their experiences with therapists who helped them to develop strategies to deal with the challenges of their new role.

Care for the Caregiver

Even though caregivers to persons with dementia have been referred to in some of the literature on the subject as the "invisible second patient," they receive very little "care" from the healthcare system. While the literature tells us that involving caregivers as partners in health care is important, it is equally important to recognize them as part of the "unit of care."

Reg's plaintive observation helps to focus on the fact that in spite of all the help that might be available to caregivers of persons living with dementia, it is a stressful and lonely journey. As he said, "The trouble with caregiving is that no one cares for you, so you don't have time for yourself ever and the person who would have taken care of you can't do it and doesn't know she can't anymore. It is such a lonely feeling."

Support from a Faith Community

Caregivers who reported having ties to a faith community gained significant support from their community and their beliefs. For example, Marion reported finding strength in the support of her church friends. Donalda also benefitted from respite care provided by members of her church. Other caregivers mentioned that members of their faith communities visited their family member while they were in long-term care.

Having an active prayer life also benefits certain caregivers. For example, Sophie suggested that, "My prayers have given me the strength and guidance I needed."

Some caregivers had an approach to life shaped by their faith and this also saw them through many of the challenges of caregiving. Donalda for instance sees her situation as "God's gift to help us be good to each other in this time, because you never know, it could be you next." Marion credits her faith as contributing to her ability to live one day at a time. Brenda said that her faith is "everything [to her]. I know who is caring for me and that allows me to care for others." She suggested that this attitude is not uncommon throughout the African Nova Scotian community. "It is part of our culture to take in everyone and by extension we want to keep family members at home and support them the best we can."

Ling said that although they are not religious *per se* they do follow Buddhist teachings and they are "important lessons for life."

Support Provided in Long-Term Care

As caregiving became too onerous a task, many caregivers chose to place the person receiving care in a long-term care facility. It is of note that sleep disturbance as well as behavioural challenges and increased physical care were typically mentioned as the rationale for placement.

It is also important to note that admission to long-term care reduced the immediate responsibility for physical care, but it did not necessarily reduce stress on the caregiver. Anne spoke of not being informed that her father had been put on medication and having to request that he be taken off. Faye spoke of the challenge of the long drive to see her husband. Loree spoke of the personhood of her father not being recognized by the care staff. And Dale spoke of the request that friends and family not visit immediately following admission to the care facility. Each of these represent factors that continue to be stressful to the caregivers.

It was the general feeling that these were examples of long-term care facilities setting up a "we–they" scenario where the caregivers were side-lined, not consulted and certainly not supported. At the same time the caregivers reported feeling guilty and anxious about the decision they had made to place the person with dementia in a long-term care facility, so they lived with a double burden — poorer quality care for the person they cared for and unease about their decision to place the individual. Due to the COVID-19 pandemic, wait times for placement into a long-term care facility has increased by 10 percent, according to an article on the CBC website titled "COVID-19 increases long-term care wait-list by 10% in Nova Scotia," written by Taryn Grant in May 2020. At that time there were more than thirteen hundred Nova Scotians on the list.

Providing Care in Times of COVID-19

As well as increasing the wait time for entry into a long-term care facility, many caregivers commented on the huge impact that COVID-19–related restrictions had on them. While a number of respondents independently described their life as a caregiver as a "roller coaster," it became even more so when restrictions were put on family visits, service delivery, visits to the doctor and program closures. COVID-19 also delayed assessments, which resulted in the delay in service provision.

Even the assessment process for services became awkward during COVID-19 restrictions. As Janet reported,

> *Having Mom sit in on the interview to be assessed for this benefit was difficult. One of the questions was "How many hours a week do you help your Mom?" I thought of all the things I do while I am with her and then the things I do for her when I may not be in her home and came up with a number. She disputed that number and I felt awkward. How can I encourage her independence and then discuss with someone right in front of her how dependent she is? They need to re-consider this assessment process for persons with dementia.*

While the rest of the world used technology to communicate with one another, persons with dementia had either not felt comfortable with this technology, were unfamiliar with it or often lost that capacity, so they totally lost touch with friends and family members. Many families reported purchasing iPads for the person being cared for but in long-term care settings there was insufficient staffing to support the regular use of technology, and as Deanna reported, even when it could be used it left her grandmother confused. "It has been really difficult because of the pandemic as none of us could visit with her and even though Mom and Dad bought her an iPad so we could Skype with her, she didn't seem to understand why we weren't there in person or sometimes even who we are."

Persons in long-term care were denied visits for months in part because of the devastating impact COVID-19 had on persons with dementia. When visits were resumed they were often very stilted, with visitors required to wear a mask and/or stay six feet away from the person they were visiting and no physical activity was allowed such as hugs or hand holding.

The Alzheimer Society of Canada (n.d.f) has acknowledged the "increased risk of severe COVID-19 disease and mortality" for persons with dementia as well as their vulnerability "to the consequences of the pandemic including containment strategies." They further recognize that "Caregivers are also strongly impacted with increased stress, anxiety and burden." To address this, the Alzheimer Society convened the COVID-19 and Dementia Task Force, compiled of leading researchers, clinicians and dementia specialists across the country, as well people with lived experience (Alzheimer Society of Canada n.d.f). The results of this task force are being posted on the Alzheimer Society of Canada website as they come in.

Palliative Care and Bereavement Support

There are very challenging issues raised by the impending death of a person with dementia. Long before dementia results in the person becoming incompetent to make decisions, it is important to discuss the individual's end-of-life requests. This might include writing advance care directives and naming a power of attorney to make medical and financial decisions when the person with dementia can no longer make them. It may also include discussing wishes with regard to organ donation, burial or cremation and end-of-life rituals. It is these types of decisions that prompted Hope to say that increased communication with her wife is "probably the best thing to come out of her illness … we talk constantly about absolutely everything — we have to, so that I know how she really is doing, and we can plan accordingly."

Palliative care services are generally available in long-term care facilities, the community and the hospital; however, the quality of this care varies. Anne for instance was shocked when her father was deemed to be "palliative" and no one in the long-term care facility told her.

Caregivers who have provided care for persons with dementia often lose contact with their social circles and are left to make the caregiving journey on their own. This is particularly true of individuals who do not have other family members. The end of this journey is traumatic and one where they could benefit from some additional support to adjust to their new reality. Amber's perspective represents that of caregivers who find themselves in this situation:

> *Some of the gals who took care of Mom through the VON did send a card after she died, but no one ever checked on me to see how I was doing or anything. It's like when the patient dies that's the end of their job or something, but they really should check on who's left now and then.*

The approach to palliative care recommended in *Dementia Strategy for Canada: Together We Aspire* addresses the need for additional caregiver support during palliative care and bereavement. The report recommends that

> palliative care can begin at the time of a dementia diagnosis and aims to reduce suffering and improve quality of life through pain and symptom management, psychological, social, emotional, spiritual and practical support, as well as support for caregivers throughout the trajectory of the condition, including after death. (Government of Canada 2018)

Many of the caregivers we interviewed spoke about dealing with the grief and loss of seeing someone they love change before their eyes throughout the dementia journey and beyond. They also spoke of the fear and the aftermath of what might happen to them after their important one dies. In this regard, the Alzheimer Society of Canada (n.d.e) suggests the following:

> Feel the pain. Allow yourself to really feel what you are feeling, no matter what that is. Denying your feelings only intensifies and prolongs the pain.
>
> Cry. Tears can be therapeutic. Let them cleanse and relieve the pain inside. Relieve tension through shouting or punching a

cushion. However, make sure that the person with dementia is safe and out of earshot or you may distress her.

Talk. Share the pain. It is important to talk about your feelings even at the most difficult times. Sharing grief will help diminish it. It can be helpful to talk to a person outside the family, such as a counsellor or trusted friend. Joining an Alzheimer Society support group gives you the opportunity to talk with others who are on a similar journey.

Keep a journal. A journal is a private place where anything can be written including unfulfilled wishes, guilt, anger and any other thoughts and feelings. A journal is a place where you can explore your frustrations and express your thoughts and ideas without interruption.

Consider your own needs. If you spend a lot of time with the person with dementia, taking regular breaks can keep you in touch with the outside world and raise your morale. Just relaxing with a cup of tea or having a good chat on the phone will help you recharge your batteries and cope with your emotions.

Find comfort. Different people have different ways of finding comfort. For many there is comfort in rituals, such as prayer, meditation or other activities.

Hold off. Tread carefully before making decisions. Thoroughly explore all options before making major steps. You may be unable to make important decisions at times.

Be kind to yourself. Be patient with your feelings. Find a balance between the happy and sad person, the angry and peaceful and the guilty and glad self. Have patience with yourself.

Learn to laugh again. Rediscover your sense of humour. Watch a funny movie, read the comics, or spend time with a friend who makes you laugh. Finding joy in life can be one way of honouring the happy times you used to share with the person with dementia.

In terms of more appropriate strategies for palliative and end-of-life care for persons with dementia, CADTH (Canadian Agency for Drugs and Technologies in Health) notes the following:

It has been reported that at the end of their lives, people with dementia may be suffering unnecessarily and not receiving adequate pain medications and other recognized palliative care interventions. They may be transferred to acute care hospitals, which are not set up to provide appropriate care for them. A Canadian study on dying in long-term care homes concluded that challenging behaviours were more common in people with dementia at the end-of-life. Because of communication difficulties, conditions such as pain and difficulty breathing may not be as readily detected in people with dementia at the end of life, and improved management of these symptoms was noted as a priority area for quality improvement. Some modifiable organizational factors were associated with improved end-of-life care, including leadership, staff engagement, and use of best practices to manage responsive behaviours non-pharmacologically. (CADTH 2019)

Pointing out that a variety of palliative and end-of-life care is required, this organization also suggests the following:

Over the past 20 to 30 years, alternative dementia care models have been developed. The shift in focus has been to better understand the needs of the person living with dementia. Meeting these needs requires changing the underlying values for the provision of care, adjusting staffing models, redesigning physical care environments, and altering care interventions.

The new models discussed above share many commonalities and are part of a broader "culture change" in nursing home care — moving away from traditional medicalized, institutional types of care for people living with dementia. The focus is on person-centred care and the idea of enabling a "life worth living." According to this website person-centred care … focuses on the individual needs of a person rather than on efficiencies of the care provider; builds upon the strengths of a person; and honors their values, choices and preferences. … [It] reorients the medical disease-dominated model of care that can be impersonal for those oriented to holistic wellbeing that encompasses all four human dimensions: bio-psycho-social-spiritual. (CADTH 2019)

We look forward to some of these innovative strategies for providing more person-centred palliative and end-of-life care for persons with dementia and their important ones.

5

Observations and Recommendations

In the final topics that we discussed in our interviews with caregivers, we asked them to identify whether or not their experiences as a caregiver had affected how they feel about themselves. We also asked what recommendations they would make to others just starting the journey of caring for or supporting someone with dementia. Finally, we asked if there were other aspects of their caregiving stories which they would like to expand on or share. Here are their responses.

Amber

One of the experiences which many caregivers shared was a loss of self after the death of their important ones. Amber phrased it this way,

> *When the end came and Mom died, I was really at a loss. I just didn't feel like me anymore; I was always known as Joeleen's kid and I felt like now I was nobody. It was like she took my heart out of me when she died. I haven't gotten over it and I doubt I ever will. It is the worst thing that ever happened to me and I miss her every day.*

When asked if she had learned anything about herself as a result of this experience, Amber replied,

> *I never realized when she was alive how much I depended on Mom, how much I loved her and how good she was to me. I wish I had told her more often what she meant to me and how proud I was to have her as my mom. I used to think I would be stronger when the end came but I just fell apart.*

While Amber did not have specific recommendations for other caregivers, it is of note that she contributed her story because she felt it was "important that people know how dreadful this disease is, how much people suffer when someone you love has it, and you never get over it really."

Annabelle

Annabelle, who lives on a reserve, spoke of her concern that families do not have appropriate housing to care for their family members and the community does not have facilities that could be used for this purpose. For example, "I made many requests for a granny suite to better support my mother as this disease progressed, but I got no support." In general, Annabelle suggested "caregivers of persons with dementia in our community lack proper funding and supports." Added to her frustration was the fact that, "Our community is right in the city and we still cannot access provincial services that are available to the greater population."

According to Annabelle, there is judgment about placing a family member in long-term care.

> Just a few weeks ago I had another community member tell me I didn't do enough for my mom and I shouldn't have placed her in a home. I would like us to address this if we could — at the very least draw attention — to the shortcomings of the current system. We need more nursing homes and trained staff on reserves so we can keep our elder's at home. It makes me angry how they treated my mother in long-term care, but if they had helped me more she would still be in my home and getting better care than anywhere else.

Anne

Anne was pleased that her father lived close to her so that she was able to support him and share that experience with her children. She said,

> Having my dad close by allowed me to bring him to my house which I did regularly. Maintaining and supporting him became a family activity that I shared with my children — it filled my mind, body and spirit. Because my father died with Alzheimer's I am paying attention to my own brain health. I am also going to complete 23 and Me [a DNA kit]. I have also learned a lot about AD [Alzheimer's disease] by seeking out information — I feel that supporting Dad has given me the lived experience diploma in AD!

Betty

Looking back on her caregiving experiences, Betty felt that her confidence had diminished and she was still feeling the same doubts about how she had handled the situation while caring for her mother. She also felt very strongly that while providing support it was "very important to find out the likes and dislikes of that person and to try and accommodate those desires when making decisions about their care." She said that a question caregivers could ask themselves to be more reflective of the person's needs is "Would I want this for myself?"

Brenda

Brenda reported that almost every day of caregiving is challenging, but every day is also a privilege.

> *Dad's situation has made me more aware of my own responses and my responsibility to others. I have found that I have strength beyond what I could have imagined, and I am doing things now that I never thought I would or could do. These are lessons I have learned caring for my dad.*
>
> *I play multiple roles — daughter, primary caregiver, chef, cab driver, nurse, housekeeper, mother, friend, sister, life coordinator. I am always tired — physically, mentally and emotionally. Knowing that support is available and that I will have a weekend break keeps me going.*

Dale

Dale learned that friendship can transcend challenges. She stated,

> *I learned that true friendship goes beyond the boundaries of age and changing ability. My journey with Peggy was informed by my faith — I believe that life has an ebb and flow, and the Spirit calls us to respond in different ways at different times. In this sense my relationship with Peggy was Spirit-led. I was driving by the LTC facility on a day that was not my scheduled day for visiting and I felt led to visit her. When I was with her, I had the feeling that I would not see her again, so I said goodbye. She died the next day.*
>
> *When she was still lucid Peggy asked me to eulogize her after*

she died. That was my last gift to my friend Peggy and was the last role I took on in our relationship.

Deanna

Deanna said that the changes in her grandmother's health and roles has changed her life in that

I really miss her; I miss talking with her and sharing my secrets with her. She was like my best friend all my life. When I had issues with my parents when I was younger, I could talk to her about it and she never told them anything. Now I feel so badly for my mom because she has lost her best friend too. She and Oma were very close. Mom doesn't share her feelings much but I know she is hurting and scared.

Deanna said that she has learned certain things about herself as a result of her grandmother's dementia.

You should never ever take anything for granted. We would never have expected this to happen to Oma — she was always so strong and smart. She kept up on all the latest news and politics, she was an avid reader and could talk to anyone about anything. You should always tell people you love that you do. I do that every day with my boyfriend and parents. I don't want them to ever forget that, even if I do one day.

When asked if she has any recommendations to share with others facing similar experiences of caring for loved ones with dementia, Deanna said,

Be sure to talk to everyone involved; find out as much as you can about the symptoms and the stages the person might go through. Don't be scared to ask questions of the doctors and nurses and try to be as supportive as you can. Even though they may not recognize you, know that they are in there somewhere and that doesn't change how much you love them, not maybe for who they are now, but who they were.

Deb and Cathy

Both women agreed that this experience of caring for someone with dementia causes them to "feel very scared that it could happen to one of us. After all they say it runs in families don't they?" Deb said, "I don't know what I would do if this happened to Cathy. I don't know who I would be without her and I am so scared of what that would be like."

The only strategies the two women could think of in terms of how to deal with the challenges of caring for someone with dementia were, as Deb said, "Make sure you have people around you to understand and help." "If you can afford to get them meals delivered then that's a big help," said Cathy. She also said that she was going to a counsellor to help her deal with her mother's illness and her own "fears that I might get it. So far she has been great."

Diane

Diane's advice is

> Patience! Patience! Patience! Do not correct what your loved one says. Be understanding of other family members; their reactions and views might be different than yours, but are valid too. Access the support of neighbours, friends, family and healthcare providers. It is important to realize that everyone in the family has a different relationship with the person with dementia, different from yours. It is a torturous journey in which you are constantly looking for solutions.

Donalda

Donalda said the she would recommend to others doing this work that they

> try to get some people to help you. Find someone to talk to about it because is can be very lonely, especially when the one with the Alzheimer's doesn't always know who you are. Try to get enough sleep too because I know when I am tired, which seems to be mostly always, I don't function as well as I should.

At the end of our interview Donalda said she wanted us to tell people that

> we should all be asking why so many are getting this disease and what is being done about it. Right now, there is no cure and not very many medications or help around the home. Here the von is

so busy and they don't have enough workers; the schools are not putting out enough CCAs and we need to tell the governments that we need more. My doctor says the numbers are going to get higher all the time, so do something now if you want better services for yourself and your older ones.

Edith

When asked if she could recommend any coping strategies that she used when providing care to Tom, Edith said,

Other than trying to get a bit of time to myself, which was very hard to do some days because he didn't like it when I wasn't there, I would say I tried to stay positive. I was lucky to have friends and family I could talk to and have a good cry with, and those things helped me cope every day.

Edith said that if she had to

have the experience again I would have put Tom in a nursing home sooner. You don't realize how much work it is to take care of them until you are doing it, and then it's too late because the system wants them to stay home and out of outside care. There are so many waiting to get into nursing homes, yet they don't really help you to manage at home. Even though there is a lot of guilt around putting your mate in a home, you have to think about your own health too, especially when you are older. I just feel very sorry for the ones who live alone and have no family to help them out. I am fortunate.

Faye

Faye learned a number of things from her caregiving experience. For one, she said that caring for Bob added to her life and she did not regret it for a minute. She became painfully aware of how little is available through the government programs and the high cost of purchasing your own services. The lack of nighttime respite care became the factor that she believes led to her becoming stressed. She found it unreasonable that she was not able to access a LTC bed closer to home and that there appeared to be no consideration for the fact that in her late eighties she would have to drive over an hour to see her husband.

The roles she filled included wife, chauffeur, kin-keeper (communicator with family), stepmother, nurse, recreation therapist and advocate. That is a lot to take on for a woman who was almost 90 and married to a man for less than three years!

Hope

In terms of caring for her wife, Hope said,

> *As difficult as it is, I think I would say two things: one, their illness is not about you, and so the hard things they may say or do are their illness talking and not the person you love, and two, their illness might not be about you, but the effects are completely about you, so take care of yourself in whatever ways work best for you. Pay other people to do things if you can, accept help if it is genuinely offered, learn what really matters and focus on those things. I gave up ironing. Now I only buy clothes that look fine coming out of the dryer.*

Jan

When asked if the experience of living with dementia has affected how she feels about herself, Jan said,

> *Definitely. I used to be a highly competent and confident woman, very politically astute and aware and an intellectual. Now I feel scared and anxious about what else I might lose as a result of this. I'm just not myself anymore. It is not a good feeling and no matter how I try I cannot shake it off.*

Jan said that she would recommend to others facing a similar journey to her own to

> *not wait if you feel that your memory is changing and you are forgetting things; it may be something simple and not Alzheimer's. The more you let the worry fester the more depressed you get, almost to the point of not functioning anymore. Tell someone, anyone, how you are feeling and don't bottle it up alone.*

Jane

In discussing what advice Jane would give to persons supporting people living with dementia, she said, "Don't try to do everything! Hope there is no COVID-19 around. Reach out for help! Make room for "time-out." If the individual makes it difficult if you take some "time off" find a way to cope or plan a strategy to deal with that behaviour. If people offer help, take it!"

Janet

When reflecting on what she has learned from her experience that might help other caregivers, Janet mused, "In order to be effective I need time alone to re-charge and I have to plan for that. I also have to realize that people are not always going to understand my mom or my choices and that is okay — I have to trust myself."

Jeff

Jeff said that he couldn't think of coping strategies that he has learned caring for Stella because

I was able to care for Steve at home before he had to go into the hospital, so I learned a bunch of stuff then which I was able to use now. I would recommend that others in the same place ask for help if they feel they need it and to not be ashamed of asking. I know some people do feel like that from talking to friends. I feel sorry for all the people going through this situation and do feel that more needs to be done for the patients and the family and friends who care for them.

John

John said that what he has learned about himself is

patience, fear, sadness and a real wanting for things to be as they were. I am scared of the future and what I will do if she gets worse and has to go into one of those nursing home places. I want her to stay at home as long as I can manage. I know none of us lives forever but I never thought this would happen to us.

Kelli

Kelli said that her coping strategies included

reading a lot of books and checking out [websites] about Alzheimer's disease. I did look at some of the chat rooms too, but I found them too depressing and a lot of people were just not getting the right information which really pissed me off. I walk a lot and would go into the woods and just let my mind wander to wherever. A friend and I would also kayak and I really enjoy being on the river. I found it comforting and relaxing. Shopping was a help too.

She also said she did not have recommendations for others in the same situation because she feels that

every situation is different and every caregiver unique. We all have our baggage when it comes to our parents and upbringing. In my experience it wouldn't have made any difference if others told me how to deal with it all; I had to learn it as I was doing it. I am a self-reflective person anyway so really had to take a hard look at myself through all of this. Not everyone can do that or learn to do it. I don't think giving advice is helpful.

Ling

In response to these questions, Ling commented that it would

be much better if Nova Scotia encouraged more Chinese business-people to come here. Then there would be more hospitals and care places knowledgeable about our ways and how we care for our older family members. When we went to the hospital with Gao, the medical staff knew nothing about China or how we do things there and we had a hard time finding a translator to explain things to her as we weren't always in the room with her. We now pay taxes to the Canadian government and we should expect that we will receive services based on our needs.

Loree

Loree found that one of the most beneficial things one can do for caregivers is to document one's records, wishes and decisions.

Having just completed sorting through my father's estate, one of the things that strikes me as most important is the need to make (and document) decisions and maintain up-to-date records for the benefit of those who must support you while you live and look after things after you die.

My father did not plan for his dementia but luckily he had planned for his eventual death and this made my job much easier. Had my father not addressed this while he was well and of sound mind it would have been a huge burden for me and my siblings. All my dad's documents were kept in a binder and included house deeds, pension documents, insurance policies, burial plot information (with contact numbers), power of attorney, advanced health care directives and bank account numbers and locations. Thank you, Dad!

Finally, as an adult orphan, I am left with the nagging question: Would the legacy of dementia my father received from his mother be my legacy too?

Marion

Marion said that the whole caregiving experience has led her to self-reflect and look at what advice she could give to others embarking on their own journey. Marion went on to suggest that each caregiver must plan to avoid burnout. She said, "It is important to talk, talk and talk some more." She noted that sleep is very important and it was only after Dick went into hospice that Marion realized how tired she was. She also mentioned she took a six-week caregivers course with the Alzheimer Society. This course was held once a week with a different speaker each week. Subjects included legal and social concerns and home care and information about different organizations that provided care and support to caregivers.

Mary

The major learning that Mary took from her experience of providing care to Max was that she had missed many small signs of mental deterioration. As a result, it was late into Max's decline that she actually got an explanation about the changes she was observing. She also experienced both the benefits and challenges of having family help with the care. Finally, she emphasized that while family and community services may be available in the daytime, it is the nighttime that is most challenging and this is when caregiving becomes a burden.

Mike

Mike is an only child engaged to an only child. In sharing his family story, he was clear the tremendous responsibility that he feels. "I am an only child, and the pressure is really heavy."

When asked what Mike has learned about himself as a result of the dementia, he replied,

> I wish there was more education and information out there about how to deal with all of this. I never got anything from the doctor or the VON and everything I learned I had to get online from the Alzheimer's Society.
>
> Really, I just see only losses and huge ones at that. Not just for Mom and Dad, but me and Kelly [Mike's fiancée] as well. Instead of planning our wedding and being really happy about our new life together, I am just freaked out about what we will do if Dad dies. Then Mom might not be able to manage on her own and we would have to come home to take care of her or have her live with us. Kell's mom is getting up there too age-wise. She is an only child too, so we could be looking at a future of providing care for both of our mothers. We have kind of decided not to try for children because we might not be able to care for them as well as our parents. That wasn't in our plans at all.

Pam

Pam said that she wishes that there was

> more information and education about this horrible disease and how to cope with it. I never knew anything about it until it happened to us and then I was at a loss as to what to do. The doctors can't tell you everything and although he [the doctor] was supportive, he wasn't there every day. I was trying to do my best, and some of the time not doing a really good job at it. I have learned not to blame myself even though I really want to — just to blame someone, you know. Let's face it, it's the pits and it seems like everyone you meet knows someone who is dealing with this.

Reg

Among the coping strategies Reg used to help him deal with his situation was to

> read a lot of books when she was napping and not needing my constant attention. It just took my mind off what was happening. I especially enjoy war stories and historical fiction. If she was asleep, I would also watch some of the old DVDs we have, even though I have seen them so many times. I like the old musicals, like Hello Dolly, Les Misérables, Fiddler on the Roof and some others.

Reg said that these experiences have changed the way he feels about himself. He said,

> I am much more lonely than I thought I would be on my own. I would be afraid sometimes of what would happen to Nell if anything happened to me. I also worry about what is going to happen to me, especially if I get sick. I don't enjoy cooking for myself and order in a lot, but I just eat because I know I have to keep up my strength. I probably drink more than I should too. Instead of just a beer on the weekend, now I sometimes have one or two in the week, just to take the edge off, you know.

Reg said that he didn't have recommendations for others in similar circumstances because "everyone is different and what works for me may not for someone else. I don't hold with telling others what to do. We all have to figure out what is best for us in our circumstances."

Sarah

Sarah credits her faith for seeing her through the challenging times. Her first husband had died at age 28, leaving her to raise two young children. She said that as she looked at his casket she had a firm conviction that "this is not the end." This unshakable belief helped her to support her mom through her final journey.

Shirley

One of the crucial coping strategies which Shirley used to help her deal with Bill's illness was *to see a therapist. When John [the caregiver] came I would see a woman in Kentville and she helped me a lot. The trouble is that when you are in their office everything seems different and you think you can cope, but then you go home and none of those strategies work when he is waking you up every hour at night and you can't sleep and are exhausted all the time. That's when you really need the help. Still if you can afford it, it really helps to talk to a stranger about how you feel, rather than to burden your family and friends who get sick of talking about it I am sure.*

When Shirley was asked if she had any advice for others in a similar situation of caring for a loved one with Alzheimer's disease or another dementia, she reiterated some of the responses she had given to some of the questions.

Try to be patient. Don't expect them to remember the past because they can't. Try not to get frustrated with them; be realistic (which I wasn't) about what you can and can't do and don't beat yourself up (which I still do) if they have to go into a nursing home. Forgive yourself for the guilt and resentment — it is the most difficult job you will ever have. See a counsellor if you can afford it; get a massage if you can afford it. Don't be afraid or ashamed to ask for help from neighbours and friends, but choose wisely so you don't feel judged by them. Don't keep asking yourself (which I do) if there was anything you could have done differently or better. At the time you have to recognize that you did the best you could in the circumstances.

At the end of the interview Shirley said that she has been having memory issues herself, and her daughter and sons have decided that she should go to live with one of them in Maine. However, due to the COVID-19 pandemic, this is not an option at present. As well she said,

I don't want to leave here; his spirit is in this house and all around me. I want to die here if I can, but I also don't want to get sick and not be able to care for myself or end up in a nursing home. I have told the children that if I get any type of dementia, I am going to ask for Medical Assistance in Dying rather than suffer the way that Bill did.

Sonia and Andy

One of the ways which Sonia was able to find coping strategies to assist her with caring for her father was through attending

> *a local support group for people who were taking care of family members with Alzheimer's and dementia. There were just the six of us — all ladies. Most were taking care of their husbands but two of us were taking care of our parents. My family doctor recommended I attend and a local woman I know was running the group. I found the group helpful but some of their stories were harder than mine so in the end I found it too depressing to keep going. Two of the ladies in the group lost their husbands to the disease and that didn't help one bit.*

Other strategies which helped included

> *listening to CDs when Dad and Andy were in bed. I like all kinds of music and songs and when I was on my own I could just relax a bit. I also read before I go to sleep at night — mostly books about the local area, and that helped me get to sleep. I often fell asleep in the middle of a book so had to go back and read sections again. A glass of wine helped now and then too.*

When Andy was asked this question, he said,

> *Sometimes I talked to Ms. Atkinson about Grandy and she loaned me a book about a little boy who helps his grandad. It was called* Albert the Fix-it Man. *I really liked that one. As well, my best friend Dylan and me would talk about Grandy and he has a grandad too, but he doesn't have anything wrong with him yet, so he couldn't really get it. I talk to Mom too, and she tells me what is happening with Grandy so that's good too.*

Sonia would recommend to others caring for someone with dementia or Alzheimer's that they

> *don't give up. There is support out there. It isn't always easy to find or get it but you can ask at the drug stores, your family doctors, the VON and other places like that. I find in my community that lots of people have family and friends with these disorders and it*

is important to know we are not alone. So be ready to reach out. I know from the group that some people are ashamed to have people in their lives with dementia. That doesn't make sense to me. So, don't be embarrassed or ashamed. One of the women in the group said that she felt discriminated against by her neighbours. This made me so mad. It isn't contagious for God's sake! I know for some this is hard, but I know I need time for myself, especially at night, so try to get some "you time."

Andy suggested that "other kids help their moms and dads too if they have one. We can do a lot of things to help and that way our grandads know we love them, just as they are now, even if they are different than they used to be. They can't help it can they?"

Sophie

Sophie approached caregiving as both a poet and a pragmatist.

My culture plays a role because it is my duty to care for our parents and in-laws, especially those who are aging, and as I did with my stepmother-in-law and parents, it is a humble privilege. You do not think about it; it is not an obligation, it's just cycles of life. I was so blessed to have had the opportunity I had to care for a loving and amazing father-in-law.

My husband and I were married in 2007. We always supported each other and made decisions together.

Sophie and her husband have experienced six deaths or serious surgeries in the family since then. "We have yet to go on a honeymoon. People thought we would be divorced by now. If anything this made us closer and stronger. Who needs a honeymoon?"

Maintaining open communication and a sense of humour also allowed Sophie to maximize support of her father-in-law. She suggested to

let the journey unfold itself. Do not fight it or the person; look at it as a railway track — the train is stuck and not sure to go left or right. Guide the person with the dementia by validating their reality and finally, humour — laugh with (not at) the person and at the disease.

Communication at all levels is so important. Ensure the person's wishes are always in their best interest. Annual family meetings are helpful and ensuring after-death wishes are important. It is also important to educate nursing home and hospital staff about your loved one.

Verline

Verline recommends that it is helpful to be open to new learning. She said,

It is important to be prepared for good and bad surprises and I have had some "happy shocks" along the way. I know that I have grown a backbone and become much more independent as a result of Frank's condition. I believe that I have found some degree of purpose in our situation — my task is to look after someone who needs me, and I am doing that and still finding balance.

Viki

Viki has found value accessing family respite support, in attending mindfulness training workshops in Halifax on a regular basis and in practising yoga and meditation.

Discussion: Observations and Recommendations

Below is a discussion about how the caregivers believe they were affected by their experience of caregiving and what they would recommend to others just starting the journey of caring for or supporting someone with dementia. The caregivers who shared their stories had a lot of accumulated wisdom.

While each of the caregivers had a unique journey, they shared many lessons learned. These include:

- reach out when you need help;
- make plans to avoid burnout;
- be prepared to learn as you go;
- expect the journey to be a lonely one;
- keep the lines of communication open with family members;
- use the resources available through the Alzheimer Society;
- realize that every caregiver journey is unique;
- expect to encounter some degree of ignorance and/or judgment;

- sleep when you can;
- be more aware of the signs of dementia;
- do end-of-life planning early on;
- make your own end-of-life plans;
- don't take your health or that of your family members for granted; and
- validate the reality of the person living with dementia.

Strategies that specific caregivers found helpful include:

- meditation and yoga;
- taking a caregiver's course;
- talking to others in the same situation;
- reading for information and/or pleasure;
- enjoying music;
- participating in a support group;
- connecting with a therapist;
- having a good cry;
- finding opportunities to laugh;
- leaning into your faith; and
- trusting your judgment.

Recommendations that the caregivers would make to government include:

- introduce more culturally responsive care;
- provide more support to manage caring at home;
- provide sufficient long-term care options close to home;
- provide access to nighttime respite care;
- train more people to provide home care;
- hire more people to provide home care;
- provide more education about dementia;
- consider family members part of the care team;
- provide bereavement services for caregivers;
- provide an option for persons living with dementia to access Medical Assistance In Dying;
- provide support for housing options that make caregiving easier; and
- build long-term care facilities on reserves.

Some of the stories reflected positive changes or discoveries in the life of the caregivers:

- "I know that I have grown a backbone and become much more independent as a result of Frank's condition."
- "I have found that I have strength beyond what I could have imagined, and I am doing things now that I never thought I would or could do. These are lessons I have learned caring for my dad."
- "Maintaining and supporting him became a family activity that I shared with my children — it filled my mind, body and spirit."
- "I have learned how to be a better daughter and even Mom."

Caregivers shared that they learned to trust their intuition and best judgment:

- "I was driving by the LTC facility on a day that was not my scheduled day for visiting and I felt lead to visit her. When I was with her I had the feeling that I would not see her again, so I said goodbye. She died the next day."
- "People are not always going to understand my mom or my choices and that is okay — I have to trust myself."
- "Don't keep asking yourself (which I do) if there was anything you could have done differently or better; at the time you have to recognize that you did the best you could in the circumstances."
- "Even though there is a lot of guilt around putting your mate in a home, you have to think about your own health too, especially when you are older."

A significant number of caregivers found that their experience resulted in fear and anxiety for the future, whether it be fear for the person for whom they are providing care or fear that they or people they love may be affected by dementia:

- "I feel very scared that it could happen to one of us, after all they say it runs in families don't they?" Deb said. "I don't know what I would do if this happened to Cathy. I don't know who I would be without her and I am so scared of what that would be like."
- "I am just freaked out about what we will do if Dad dies. Then Mom

might not be able to manage on her own."

- "I am left with the nagging question: Would the legacy of dementia my father received from his mother be my legacy too?"
- "Now I feel scared and anxious about what else I might lose as a result of this and I'm just not myself anymore."

Caregivers found it helpful to remember who the person they are caring for was as well as who they are now:

- "Even though they may not recognize you, know that they are in there somewhere and that doesn't change how much you love them, not maybe for who they are now, but who they were."
- "The hard things they may say or do are their illness talking and not the person you love."
- Andy suggested that "other kids help their moms and dads too, if they have one. We can do a lot of things to help and that way our grandads know we love them just as they are now, even if they are different than they used to be. They can't help it can they?"

This theme emerged again in follow-up discussions with caregivers. One in particular noted that after the death of his wife who had dementia, people who were offering consolation focused on what she was like just before death and failed to acknowledge the full life she had lived before developing dementia. He pointed out, "I mourned the losses brought on by dementia a long time ago, but I was grieving a deep loss at the time of her death for the person my wife was before dementia."

A recent study of primary family caregivers supporting persons with dementia highlights the different approaches to caregiving (Leggett, Bugajski, Gitlin and Kales 2021). After studying one hundred caregivers who had provided care for an average of fifty-five months and represented a range of ages, relationships and cultural backgrounds, five "management styles" emerged. These included the following:

- "Externalizers" — superficial understanding, self-focused, frequently expressing expressions of anger or frustration.
- "Individualists" — provide care by going it alone, emotionally removed and lack management strategies.
- "Learners" — recognize the need to change their approach but are

stuck and emotionally turbulent.

- "Nurturers" — positive affect and empathy toward care and natural mastery.
- "Adapters" — had an arsenal of acquired management strategies and adapt to challenges.

The researchers found that the styles differed in terms of age and use of formal supports.

While these may reflect in whole, in part or in a combination of styles the caregivers we interviewed, we contend that the stories we collected generally reveal a more nuanced picture of caregiving — one that is committed, reflective and flexible. The caregivers who shared their experiences found that theirs was a journey they navigated on their own terms, learning from each new day and each new circumstance. Their caregiving was a work in progress and as one caregiver said, "I had to learn it as I was doing it."

In an attempt to determine what contributes to the resilience of the caregivers we interviewed, we looked at a study that reviewed forty-six peer-reviewed articles on the subject published between 1990 and 2018 (Zhou, O'Hara, Ishado, Borson and Sadak 2019). The authors found that the following factors contributed to resiliency in caregiving provided to persons with dementia:

- engaging in problem identification and problem solving;
- self-growth behaviours including self-care, creative/spiritual activities and developing and/or maintaining meaningful social relationships; and
- the willingness to seek out and receive help.

The narratives we collected reflect that many of the caregivers were learning the value of these resiliency strategies and incorporating them into their caregiving role and their personal lives where possible.

The caregivers offered a number of observations sprinkled throughout their stories which were not specifically addressed by our interview questions. These included observations about

- feeling blindsided by the diagnosis of dementia;
- the necessity to support the reality of the person living with dementia;

- the impact of poor financial judgment;
- the effects of dementia on romantic relationship; and
- the judgment of the caregiver's actions.

Caregivers referenced the arrival of dementia in their lives as a surprise that blindsided them in the following comments:

- "I thought her mood swings and memory loss were the result of the medications they had her on."
- "I assumed it was because he was going through missing work and the role he played there."
- "We figured it was because she missed Tyrone [her husband] and was still grieving."
- "We (the family) did not consider dementia. Perhaps because there was no history of dementia in our family, or that we were more focused on my mother and her health issues."
- "She thought it was Peggy's age or maybe fatigue that was affecting her."
- "We never knew if what we observed was the effects of dementia or alcohol."
- "We were in denial because she was so young."

Dr. Samir Sinha, director of Health Policy Research at the National Institute on Ageing at Ryerson University in Toronto points out that dementia is much more than memory loss. It can appear as spatial disorientation, mood changes, withdrawal or a decrease in problem solving skills among other changes in abilities or personality.

He also suggests that there are other issues that may account for many of what are classic signs of dementia. Hearing loss, medications, mental health issues or other illnesses may appear to be dementia. For these reasons families can be surprised by the diagnosis of dementia (RBC Wealth Management n.d.).

The value in living with the reality of the person with dementia was discussed by caregivers in the following ways:

- One thing that Janet struggles with is not being honest with her mother. Honesty and integrity were values her mother taught her and it seems duplicitous to use approaches that require her to lie.

On the other hand, she knows better than to confront her mother's reality. She finds that although her mother may get confused about the literal content of a conversation, she is often accurate as to the emotional content and this can affect her.

- "We just treated her as if her perception of the world was the truth; there was no sense in arguing."
- This helper insisted that Max live in the "real world." If it was Monday and Max said it was Tuesday he was shown the error of his ways. If this approach of focusing on dates, locations and names were woven into the conversations with Max it might have been helpful, but the constant correcting by this caregiver was more than Mary could handle.

A resource on communication from the *Day To Day* series available through the Alzheimer Society of Canada provides the following advice on living with the reality of the person with dementia:

> With the progression of the disease, a person's perception of reality can become confused. However, it is their reality. Try to accept their reality and meet them where they are. Avoid contradicting them or convincing them that what they believe is untrue or inaccurate. Trying to bring them into your reality or disagreeing with them will cause frustration and make things worse. If they say something you know isn't true, try to find creative ways around the situation rather than reacting negatively. (Alzheimer Society of Canada n.d.a)

The loss of household money as a result of poor judgment exercised by the person with dementia was raised as a concern by a number of caregivers:

- "The caregiver started calling every day with stories about things that Malcom was doing — giving away money, telling people his credit card numbers and driving."
- "I asked to see the correspondence regarding this purchase and found that the firm had promised to print and market the books for a ridiculously high price, which my father had paid. He knew that he had got in over his head and did not know how to get out. It was sad to see his hard earned dollars be used to line the pockets of

unscrupulous people who clearly preyed on those who were unable to look after their own best interests."

- One of the challenges that Verline faces is that Frank lost all their retirement income before she took over the finances. As a result, money would be an issue if Frank were institutionalized. The partner who resides in the community gets only a portion of the resident's pension, and Verline said that this would not leave her enough to maintain the home.

The vulnerability of persons with dementia to schemes to defraud them is a subject that is being increasingly documented. In an article by Carol Cohen from the University of Toronto as part of the Dementia Series, it is highlighted that

> individuals who are successfully defrauded often cannot understand or appreciate this fact because of cognitive impairment. They cannot grasp the connection between their actions — sending money to claim fake lottery winnings, and the outcome — loss of these funds and no prize earnings. By the time family and friends realize what is going on, losses may be extensive. Dementia clinics are also reporting that being a victim of fraud has become a trigger for referral, as families realize that the senior is not processing information as they would have in the past. (Cohen 2008: 284)

The challenges of maintaining romantic, intimate relationships when caring for someone living with dementia were noted in the following discussions:

- "Even though I live with a person who looks like a man, my life as a 'woman' has ended, and I get sad about that."
- Laura also feels the effects of a husband who does not understand his role in deepening or even maintaining their relationship.
- "You aren't a wife anymore, you are some type of caretaker and it really changes your perspective on how you see yourself."
- "I miss her telling me she loves me. You know, I know somewhere in there she does, but we used to say it every day before we went to sleep, and I wish I could hear it again."
- "Because of the Alzheimer's disease and the medications he was on,

we were no longer intimate and sometimes he was very aggressive and behaved inappropriately in terms of trying to grab or fondle me or say nasty sexual things. I know it wasn't him but the disease."

- "I was a single woman who could not think about a new relationship because my available time was consumed with my father. In the eight years between my mom's death and my dad's death my only relationship was a long distance one where I could control the time it took."

- "As Dad's dementia progressed, I no longer wanted to winter in Arizona. I felt guilty leaving my mother, even though my sister was here, and my mother wanted me to go. I felt torn between my husband's need to go away, and my need to stay in Nova Scotia to care for my family."

While romance, feeling loved and sexual intimacy remains important as people age, it can be very challenging for the partner who is providing care. While the person they love is physically present, they are experienced as a different person by the caregiving partner. The Alzheimer Society of Canada provides some insights into this aspect of the dementia journey in an online section entitled, "How your intimate relationships can change" (Alzheimer Society of Canada n.d.b).

The last two caregiver quotes in this section speak to the challenge that adult children who are providing care to parents face in their relationships. In one case, the caregiver indicates that for eight years she put on hold the possibility of developing a relationship while she looked after her dad.

The second quote from an adult child caring for her parents indicates the tension that can happen in a relationship when one partner wants to focus on what they perceive to be their caregiver responsibilities while the partner wants to continue the life pattern that was established before caregiving entered their lives.

The judgment expressed by others as the caregivers fulfilled their caregiving roles was reflected in the following:

- "A neighbour contacted Adult Protection because my father-in-law told her he was going to jump off the wharf (she did not discuss anything with us). Adult Protection suddenly arrived and acted very quickly."
- She was told she was selfish to put her mother in a nursing home,

but no one offered to help her.

- "There is a lot of social pressure and people offer their suggestions about what I should be doing."
- She said that she communicated with them (her brothers) about every change in care and she had to argue with them constantly to justify her decisions, especially when it involved the expenditure of money.
- "Just a few week ago I had another community member tell me I didn't do enough for my mom and I shouldn't have placed her in a home."

Providing care is stressful enough without being criticized for the decisions that have to be made to best support an individual living with dementia; however, judgment can be hard to avoid. The Home Care Assistance program (Hodge 2020) in Vancouver, British Columbia, offered four approaches one might use when being judged:

- Acknowledge the emotions that the criticism evokes and then move on.
- Consider the source of the criticism and attempt to identify the motivation.
- Use the remarks to open up a constructive dialogue.
- Use the comments as a way to determine whether you might benefit from increased help.

6

Closing the Gap

When we think about closing a gap, we are typically referring to reducing a difference. It might be a difference between people, ideas, policies, perceptions or groups. In this chapter we are going to explore ways in which "gaps" are being addressed in the field of dementia care.

The Gap in Research Addressing the Impact of Race and Ethnicity on Dementia Care

Because we were unable to interview as many African Nova Scotian and Indigenous people as we had planned, we conducted a literature search on this topic. We found that scant information on this subject is available from a Canadian perspective. Indeed the Alzheimer Society of Canada speaks to this gap in their October 5, 2020, statement entitled "Race and Dementia":

> At the Alzheimer Society of Canada, we work to change the lives of those living with dementia. We acknowledge that we have not done enough to combat the systemic oppression felt by Black Canadians, and how they, Indigenous Peoples and other People of Colour connect with the health services in our country. Based on information collected from the US & UK, dementia impacts Black people at higher rates with some studies showing twice the occurrence than white populations. Yet we do not know the impact this disease has on Black, Indigenous Peoples and other Canadians of colour, because the available data is minimal at best. (Alzheimer Society of Canada 2020)

Recognizing that systemic racism is part of the Canadian experience and that it contributes to the information gap, the Alzheimer Society of

Canada created an action plan which will result in an advisory group of individuals representing peoples of different races and levels of expertise who will advise future actions to remedy the situation. As well, the Alzheimer Society of Canada will conduct a national survey asking for Canadians from diverse ethnic and racial backgrounds for their experiences dealing with dementia. The material gathered from this exercise will then be shared with physicians and others providing care to persons with dementia in Canada (Alzheimer Society of Canada n.d.c).

The Alzheimer Society of Nova Scotia (2020) did produce a pamphlet on September 24, 2020, on the subject of "Dementia and People of African Descent," and in it they recognized that research shows that people of African descent are

- two times more likely to develop Alzheimer's disease and other dementia compared to Caucasians; and
- more likely to have vascular disease (problems with blood circulation) and may also be at risk for developing Alzheimer's disease and vascular dementia.

The pamphlet, intended to be used in workshops in the HRM area of the province went on to say that based on American studies, some of the risk factors for developing dementia associated with having African ancestry may be

- woman, 65 years old, has the APOE E4 AND ABCD7 gene;
- family history;
- high blood pressure;
- high cholesterol levels;
- type 2 diabetes;
- obesity;
- low education;
- living in rural areas;
- smoking;
- sedentary lifestyle; and
- heart problems.

The pamphlet was sent to us by the manager of program development from the Alzheimer Society of Canada. It is now available on their website (Alzheimer Society of Canada 2020).

While the literature on dementia among African Canadians is limited, there is more dealing with dementia among Indigenous Peoples of Canada, thanks in part to organizations such as the National Collaborating Centre for Indigenous Health, located at the University of Northern British Columbia in Prince George. Their 2018 report, authored by Julia Petrasek MacDonald, Valerie Ward and Regine Halseth, is titled *Alzheimer's Disease and Related Dementias in Indigenous Populations in Canada: Prevalence and Risk Factors*. The authors suggest, as does the organization just mentioned, that "there is a paucity of epidemiological research on ADRDs (Alzheimer's disease and related dementias) related to Indigenous people in Canada" (2018: 9). They present a list of studies conducted in provinces in Canada with larger populations of Indigenous persons than the Atlantic region, especially in Manitoba, British Columbia and Alberta, and note that based on these studies the rates of ADRDs are "expected to increase by 4.2 times for First Nations and 3.3 times for Inuit between 2006 and 2031" (2018: 9). As well, the authors point out that the onset of dementia appears to be at a younger age in Indigenous people compared to the general population.

Many of the risk factors associated with dementia among Indigenous persons mirror those from African Nova Scotians: high rates of poverty, lack of educational resources and opportunities, lack of potable drinking water, lack of employment opportunities and lack of access to health resources within specific communities. There are also those risk factors stemming from colonization and racism, the results of which are poverty, intergenerational trauma brought about from the residential school practices and the "sixties scoop," which occurred in Canada between the late 1950s and into the 1980s, when Indigenous children were taken from their families and communities or "scooped up" to be placed in foster homes or adopted by white families. The authors of this report highlight the need for "integrated multi-sectoral approaches to address the socio-economic inequities and health disparities Indigenous people are experiencing in order to stave off the potential for a dementia 'epidemic' among this population" (2018: 23).

As with the research on the impact of race and ethnicity on persons with dementia, there is also a scarcity of material which addresses the topic of the impact of these identities on caregivers of persons with dementia. In a 2013 article, published in the *Indian Journal of Gerontology*, Canadian authors McCleary and Blain examine, among other topics, the inter-related concepts of familism and filial piety. Familism, they state, "refers to strong identification and solidarity of individuals with their family as well as strong normative feelings of allegiance, dedication, reciprocity, and attachment to their family members, both nuclear and extended" (2013: 182). The authors state further: "The subcomponents of familism are: family obligation (the obligation to provide caregiving for family members); support from the family (expectation of support from family members when needed); and family as referents (rules about how life should be lived derived from the family)" (2013: 182). The concept of familism is seen to be prominent in more traditional Chinese families, but as younger people aspire to the Western notion if individualism, this is becoming less prevalent.

The above authors define filial piety as "a fundamental value in Confucian ethics that requires respect for parents and placing family needs over individual needs. It involves concern for parental health, financially supporting parents, fulfilling the housing needs of parents and respect for parental authority" (2013: 182). As McCleary and Blain point out, the concept of filial piety is most common in South Asian countries and communities, and in our interviews both Sophia and Ling spoke to this culturally accepted idea and expectation. The authors suggest that where filial piety is visible in Western cultures, it is seen to include reverence for parents; gratitude and repaying a debt of gratitude to parents for their care; and expressing love and friendship for parents through care (2013: 182).

McCleary and Blain also conducted a review of the literature on the impact of race and ethnicity on caregivers, and while recognizing that such material was in short supply, did note that "Research that compared caregivers based on their ethnic background or race found that ethnic minority caregivers tend to use less formal supports and may delay help-seeking early in the course of dementia" (2013: 189). This is a problematic finding in relation to provinces like Nova Scotia where there is a lack in some communities of specific ethnic groups, especially as Ling pointed out in her interview, when it comes to Chinese persons. Clearly where there are larger numbers of persons within a community of a specific ethnicity or culture, then more social supports are in place, as was somewhat evidenced in Donalda's, Deb's and Cathy's and Brenda's interviews.

In their conclusions to this interesting paper, McCleary and Blain state:

> There is a small but growing body of literature about the role of

cultural values in caregiving. Like previous caregiving research, most of this research tests various aspects of a stress, coping and adaptation theoretical model of family caregiving. By examining cultural values such as filial piety and familism within and across various ethnic groups, this research is beginning to bring a more nuanced understanding of the role of cultural values in the process of caregiving. (2013: 196)

We are heartened that there appears to be a commitment to closing the gap in research addressing the impact of race and ethnicity on dementia care.

The Gap in Culturally Relevant and Sensitive Care for Persons with Dementia

While the National Collaborating Centre for Indigenous Health and the Alzheimer Society of Nova Scotia are attempting to update their services for ethnically and culturally diverse clients, they do not discuss the need for culturally relevant and sensitive care for persons with dementia. Another 2018 report from the National Collaborating Centre for Indigenous Health, written by Regine Halseth and titled *Overcoming Barriers to Culturally Safe and Appropriate Dementia Care Services and Supports for Indigenous Peoples in Canada*, provides a set of strategies to meet these goals, which could apply to any ethnic or cultural group in Canada. The following are some of the strategies that Halseth (2018: 16–19) suggests:

- fostering health and supportive family and community environments;
- building local capacity through education;
- selecting strategies, programs and services to ensure quality of life;
- reducing health system barriers to dementia care services and supports; and
- creating better and more sufficient supports for caregivers.

In the first strategy — fostering health and supportive family and community environments — Halseth states that, when it comes to Indigenous Peoples, and we would argue any community, it is important to have an "understanding of how populations perceive aging well, it is important for understanding their health, healing and wellness needs" (2018: 12). Further Halseth notes:

> History, culture and language also provide the foundation for cognitive and physical stimulation, which plays a role in improving quality of life for dementia patients and preventing age-related cognitive decline and neurodegenerative diseases. The types of interventions or strategies that might contribute to a healthier and supportive family and community environment are wide-ranging. They might include strategies or initiatives that: address poverty and socio-economic marginalization within Indigenous communities; help reduce the stigma and fear of dementias and build local care capacity; aim to improve mental health and wellness within communities; encourage youth to stay in their communities; support the ability of individuals with dementia to remain in their homes with the support of families and communities for as long as they can; and provide opportunities for social, mental and physical stimulation. (2018: 12)

In the second strategy — building local capacity through education — Halseth suggests that community-based education may prove helpful and that

> reducing or eliminating the fear and stigma associated with dementias in Indigenous communities could help strengthen the process of accessing dementia care and build local capacity to deliver formal dementia care and support informal caregivers. Fear and stigma may prevent individuals from seeking an assessment, delaying appropriate care, as well as inhibit the development of community awareness of dementia and the sharing of knowledge about ways to cope with it. (2018: 18)

In the third strategy — strategies, programs and services to ensure quality of life — Halseth points out that even though the age-friendly community initiatives were created in thirty-six different cities across Canada, the specific needs of seniors from Indigenous and other ethnic and culturally diverse groups were not targeted. Neither were those living in rural or remote areas of the country. In the case of Indigenous seniors, Halseth recommends that such services and programs may include those that promote social interaction to ward off loneliness, such as support groups, community groups and other initiatives to get Indigenous seniors out of the house and away from the television. It may also include programs and services which promote mental and physical stimulation, including "supports that encourage and enable [Indigenous] seniors to participate in activities that reflect their cultural values or traditional ways of life." (2018: 19)

For the fourth category — reducing health system barriers to dementia care services and supports — Halseth discusses the need to recognize that as dementia symptoms worsen, interactions with the healthcare system become more frequent. In order to optimize the quality of care and quality of life of Indigenous people with dementia, innovation and flexibility are required to address unique barriers they face in accessing health care. Some of the innovations Halseth addresses are jurisdictional and bureaucratic considerations that may present barriers to accessing dementia care services and supports.

This includes who pays for services if they are accessed off-reserve; the lack of programs and services available for Métis and non-status Indians that are available to First Nations on reserve and Inuit, like home care and continuing support programs; as well as delays or denied approvals for medicine, supplies and medical travel due to underfunding, excessive restrictions and highly bureaucratic processes. (2018: 21)

These barriers were also addressed by Annabel in her interview.

In the fifth category — supporting caregivers — Halseth suggests

There is a need for better and more consistent supports and resources for caregivers and care recipients to address challenges associated with an outmigration of youth to urban centres, resulting in fewer family caregivers, as well as limited caregiving resources and caregiver burnout. (2018: 19)

The above recommendation mirrors feedback we heard from caregivers living in all parts of rural Nova Scotia. Like Indigenous people, those who have lived in rural areas for generations have a strong connection to place and do not want to leave the land that is their source of strength and resilience in order to access caregivers or services in other places.

Another approach recommended in the report is the consideration of shared caregiving and multi-collaborative approaches to address the current lack of access to health programs, services and resources. Collaboration would involve shared caregiving approaches where resources are pooled between families, healthcare providers and community services to meet the needs of persons with dementia and those caring for them. This report could act as a toolkit for any ethnic or racially disenfranchised group of Canadians who are attempting to receive and participate in changes to dementia in Canada. For an international approach to this topic, the Alzheimer's Society of the United Kingdom, admittedly dealing with a much larger community of different cultures and ethnic backgrounds than Canada, provides programming to address these issues on their website. They suggest that healthcare providers involve people with living with dementia, carers and target diverse communities in providing ideas and offering feedback.

> Ask them if there are food and drink or social activity traditions associated with getting together (such as dominoes, drumming, singing or doing craft activities) which you might want to integrate into your activity to make it feel welcoming and attuned to people's needs.
>
> Find out about interpreters who speak, or sign, in community languages used by people you want to engage. Find out about religious and cultural occasions which might be relevant considerations to avoid major involvement events clashing with times people are fasting, for example. (Alzheimer's Society of the United Kingdom n.d.a)

The issue of cultural sensitivity when dealing with persons with dementia is one that will need to be addressed more fully in Nova Scotia, nationally and globally as the number of cases continues to grow everywhere in the world. Fortunately, both the Alzheimer Society of Nova Scotia and the Canadian organization have made a commitment to further research these topics in order to close this gap. As a founding member and partner of the Canadian Consortium on Neurodegeneration in Aging (CCNA) that includes over 350 researchers across the country that aim to accelerate progress in the research of Alzheimer's disease, the Alzheimer Society of Canada committed $4.05 million from 2014–2019 to fund this research, which includes an examination of culturally appropriate care

(Government of Canada 2019).

Along with the need to provide accurate, culturally sensitive care to Indigenous Peoples and those from African Canadian cultures, it is also necessary to include the care which is provided to immigrants, refugees and their families, especially those providing care to important ones, as Ling pointed out, and as Deanna discussed when speaking of the ways in which her grandmother relived her experiences as a Dutch immigrant to Canada many years ago.

In a CBC News article posted online on August 25, 2020, author Olivia Bowden points out that exposing older persons with dementia (especially those in long-term care facilities) to language, food and customs they know can delay the progress of the disease. Citing the experience of a worker in a facility in Ottawa, Bowden notes:

> Zeba Taj would often come home sobbing after a shift at the long-term care home in Ottawa where she worked for three years. Many of the residents there had dementia, and many were from diverse cultural backgrounds. What upset Taj was that the elderly men and women had virtually no access to the languages, food or religious customs they'd been used to their whole lives. "They don't understand any of their activities. The one thing they know is that this is not their home," said Taj, who quit in 2017. Once, she had to insist to her supervisor that a Muslim resident who had dementia not be fed pork. "I felt so sad for this person. He doesn't know the language, food is not of his choice and he's completely isolated," said Taj, who now runs programming for seniors at the non-profit Social Planning Council of Ottawa (SPCO). (Bowden 2020)

Bowden further suggests that

> immigrant families struggle to access resources that fit their specific cultural and religious needs. Doctors often don't speak their language, nor do they always understand the stigma around dementia that exists within some ethnic communities. Close to 70 percent of residents in long-term care have dementia, according to 2016 report from the Canadian Institute for Health Information. Often, those facilities lack any culturally relevant care: residents aren't served the food they've eaten their whole lives, there's no

diverse religious or cultural programming for them and staff often don't speak their first language. If the people who are in a given long-term care facility have no commonality of life experience, it's a hugely isolating place to be.

Because family doctors and others in the health fields may not share languages with immigrants and refugees with dementia or have an understanding of their cultural values around health and wellness, the levels of care being able to be provided are complicated by these issues, as they are with any minority racial and ethnic groups. In both the Canadian and Nova Scotia dementia strategies it is noted that culturally accurate and sensitive dementia care should be recognized and that staff need to be educated on cross-cultural issues. It is our hope that increased education and the allocation of additional resources will start to close the gap and result in care that is targeted to meet the cultural needs of different groups of older persons and their caregivers.

The Gap in Care Facilities

Caregivers we interviewed were frustrated by the gaps they found in care facilities for persons with dementia. These frustrations included the need at times for persons living with dementia to be admitted to hospital in order to access a long-term care bed. Some also reported being frustrated by the distance they had to drive to get to the long-term care facility. This is further complicated in rural areas if the visiting caregiver was unable to drive or concerned about winter driving conditions. Finally, caregivers were concerned about the quality of care the person with dementia received in long-term care. They suggested that this was due in part to restrictive policies, a limited number of single rooms and insufficient staffing.

Changes Required in Long-term Care Facilities

While this book was being written, the need for improvements in care and living arrangements for older persons living in long-term care facilities in Canada became very obvious. At that time 80 percent of COVID-19 deaths in Canada occurred in long-term care facilities. This is twice as many as in other OECD countries. As a result of the obvious gaps between optimum care and what is currently being delivered in many facilities in Canada, the Elder Law Section of the Canadian Bar Association made a resolution urging the federal government to improve long-term care and support for older Canadians. Specifically, it wants to fast-track national quality standards, create pan-Canadian strategies for long-term care and elder abuse, improve infection prevention and control in long-term care, provide better assistance to caregivers and create a pan-Canadian disaster response for seniors (Pellerin 2021).

While long-term care is a provincial responsibility, CanAge, an organization which works to improve the lives of older adults through advocacy, policy and community engagement, supports the resolution. They contend that the *Canada Health Act* (CHA) has been eroded over the years, particularly for seniors, and the result is that "approximately 30% of Canadian health expenditures are now paid outside of public sources, placing Canada below the OECD average. CanAge perceives the intention behind the resolution is to restore the original purpose of the CHA" (Pellerin 2021).

In late January of 2021, the then-premier of Nova Scotia, Stephen MacNeil, announced a plan to add 226 long-term care beds in the central health zone and replace hundreds of others across the province. The potential positive impact of this infusion of funding was highlighted by Menna MacIsaac, Grand View Manor's CEO, who said rooms at the long-term care facility where she is the administrator are being shared by between two and four people and are smaller than what the current standards dictate for single rooms.

> "Often there isn't enough room for a family member to have a chair and visit," MacIsaac said. "More significantly is that a lot of the people who are in our residence are more acutely ill, and as they become palliative, families are expected to be in the same room with their loved one in a shared accommodation." In this situation, MacIsaac says that "privacy and dignity are as much an issue as infection control." (Willick 2021)

Before COVID-19 pointed out the challenges in long-term care they were clearly on the radar of the Nova Scotia Nurses' Union. In 2015 they published a report entitled *Broken Homes* in which they stated:

> Long-term care (LTC) is in desperate need of resuscitation in order to prepare for the imminent and expansive growth in our seniors population. Our system is dangerously out of step with

the times, desperately trying to keep pace but suffering from widespread malaise and neglect. An immediate, multi-pronged approach is required to remedy the litany of current and critical ailments within the sector. (Curry 2015)

In 2018 the Department of Health in Nova Scotia appointed a panel of three experts — Dr. Janice Keefe, Dr. Cheryl Smith and Dr. Greg Archibald — to review the staffing at long-term care facilities to address "overstressed" homes that aren't capable of meeting residents' needs. The panel completed their work in December and reported their findings in January 2019. The first recommendation was to "Invest in Human Resource Capacity and Enhance Staff Mix." The description of what they heard bears out this recommendation:

> Quality of care of residents in LTC facilities is affected by the quality of work life for staff. Sufficient and appropriate staffing is necessary to meet the increasing care needs of residents. We heard over and over from residents and their families that staff do not have the time to provide appropriate care because they are "working short." Shortages increase staff responsibilities, with more residents to provide care for, resulting in overstressed staff, high rates of injury and sickness and many unfilled vacancies across the sector. It was most profound to hear from staff and many of the sector representatives about the guilt and shame they feel not being able to provide adequate care. These challenges highlight the urgency to invest in human resources to alleviate the unsustainable workload and untenable physical and mental fatigue of staff. (Keefe, Smith and Archibald 2018: 6)

In spite of the recommendations made in this comprehensive report, the unions representing those working in long-term care facilities in Nova Scotia addressed the standing committee on health in January 2021, sharing their ongoing frustrations about staffing and offering recommendations on ways to improve long-term care (Guye 2021).

It is clear that the concerns raised by the caregivers we interviewed are valid, and while the additional long-term care beds in Nova Scotia will help to relieve some of the challenges in the not-too-distant future, gaps will remain until there is more movement in the identified staffing issues.

Dementia Villages

Dementia villages represent an emerging approach for providing residential long-term care, especially for people living with advanced dementia. Dementia villages share some common elements with other innovative models of residential care that emphasize improving quality of life for people with dementia by providing person-centred care in smaller scale, less institutional and more "homelike" environments.

Such facilities are normally situated within neighbourhoods but are self contained. They include all of the amenities of a town or village such as shops, banks, healthcare provider offices, hairdressers and barbers and cafés or restaurants. The major elements in the planning of Dementia Villages include:

> Design of the physical environment to accommodate the needs of people living with dementia, small-scale, home-like group living to encourage social interaction and participation in activities of daily life, ready access to outdoor space and gardens. Ensuring all residents with advanced dementia are able to participate in the activities of daily life in dementia villages, additional staff are needed. (CADTH 2019)

The first dementia village, De Hogeweyk, was developed in the Netherlands and opened in 2009. It is equipped with townhouse units that are shared by small groups of residents with similar lifestyles and interests. All the services of a small village are available to residents, like a supermarket, restaurant, pub and theatre. These design elements allow residents to live life and receive care in a more homelike setting. Person-centred care practices are applied at De Hogeweyk, with a focus on meeting the individual needs of residents while honouring their values, choices and preferences. Assisted when necessary by staff, volunteers or family, residents participate in everyday activities that are meaningful to them, like preparing meals, enjoying the garden or attending a concert. Residents remain at De Hogeweyk until they die, being supported by a palliative care team in their final days.

As well as the Netherlands and Holland, dementia villages now exist, or are in the planning stages, in many other parts of Europe, including Denmark, England, France, Germany, Ireland, Switzerland and Wales, as well as Australia and New Zealand, and in North America in the United States and Canada. The first one in Canada was being built in Langley,

British Columbia, in July 2019. In the article "A Look Inside: Canada's First 'Dementia Village,'" written by Eric Zimmer for the publication *The Daily Hive*, the journalist notes:

> Situated on the site of a former elementary school (closed in 2007), the five-acre, privately-funded community takes its inspiration from the world's first Dementia Village, *de Hogeweyk*, located in Holland, and from the *Green House Project* in the US.
> The property features six, fully-staffed, single-story cottages which can accommodate 12 people each, for a total of 72 residents.
> The cottages themselves have been designed to be [sic] offer the feel and appearance of a "normal" home. The cottages themselves are centred on a Village Plaza and Community Centre that is designed to be the activity hub of the community. (Zimmer 2019)

The Village, as this facility is known, is similar to the one in the Netherlands as it too includes

> a "general store," where residents can come for items such as small household supplies, snacks and other goods. The items are all provided free of charge, as the goal of the store is to give the residents the familiar experience of "shopping" for items themselves. The Village also features an on-site salon, workshop, medical clinic and art space. Outdoor activities are encouraged too, and residents can choose from different ideas including visiting a barn (complete with animals), a veggie patch, activity lawns, water gardens, "sensory gardens" and numerous pathways. (Zimmer 2019)

An examination on the website of The Village shows that it is an expensive option of care and therefore would limit who could afford to live there. For example, the site notes that the Base Rate does include all Village services and support such as "meals, laundry service and assistance with bathing and medication. The Complex Care Rate includes all of the elements in the Base Rate, along with more advanced 24/7 nursing care" (The Village n.d.). Items that are not included in the rates just mentioned are those such as personal expenses like toiletries and medications.

CADTH is an independent, not-for-profit organization responsible for providing Canada's healthcare decision makers with objective evidence to help make informed decisions about the optimal use of drugs and medical devices in our healthcare system. CADTH (2019) produced a report entitled *Dementia Villages: Innovative Residential Care for People with Dementia*, and concluded the following:

- Although further research and evaluation are needed, dementia villages based on the Hogeweyk Care Concept may have a place within the continuum of dementia care in Canada.
- Built environment (e.g., creating homelike environments with access to outdoor and common spaces) and living environment (e.g., encouraging social activity and meaningful participation in daily household activities) characteristics should be considered when developing or funding residential care facilities for individuals with advanced dementia.
- Before adopting new design standards or models for residential care, decision makers should consider the ease with which Canadians can access dementia villages. For example, high monthly costs for residents in private facilities, limited availability for publicly funded spots and limited accessibility for those living in rural or remote communities could make it hard for many Canadians to access dementia villages.

As this book was being written we could find no other examples of Canadian dementia villages other than the one (The Village) in Langley, British Columbia. We hope that there will be more to come as this concept appears to fill a need for more housing/support options for persons living with dementia.

Memory Care Facilities

Another concept for residential care for persons with dementia is that of memory care facilities, which are normally a form of senior living that provides intensive, specialized care for people with memory issues. Many assisted living facilities and nursing homes have created special memory care units for dementia patients. While these units were initially part of a complex within nursing homes, there are also stand-alone memory care facilities built close to the nursing home. Memory care facilities aim to empower seniors who have memory loss to stay as active and engaged as they possibly can, while living in a dignified, safe and secure setting. Many nursing homes and assisted living complexes in Nova Scotia offer memory care facilities, such as those provided by the Shannex corporation, Milestone Communities, The Parkland complexes and many others. A list of memory care facilities can be found at the Government of Nova Scotia's Ministry of Health and Wellness website (Nova Scotia Department of Health and Wellness 2021).

Transition Support

In the province of Ontario, the Ontario Shores Centre for Mental Health Sciences understands that the impact of dementia and the experience of caregiving may be

> challenging for a caregiver. The inter-professional team hopes to provide ongoing support to caregivers throughout a patient's stay at Ontario Shores. This may occur in family meetings with the inter-professional care team, special events on the unit and in referrals to supportive services, such as our Family Resource Centre.
>
> An admission to our unit(s) is expected to be temporary for stabilization and a plan for transitioning to the most appropriate setting will be established early on. Caregivers are involved in the transition process through family meetings, regular updates with the social worker and pre-discharge conferences. Outpatient services may be provided by Ontario Shores or another community provider or in collaboration together. Ontario Shores encourages caregivers to be involved in the discharge planning process as early as possible. (Ontario Shores Centre for Mental Health Sciences n.d.)

While the caregiver is encouraged to spend time in the Ontario Shores unit, for a fee, the agency ensures that their professional staff care for the person with dementia either in the same unit or in a hospital or nursing home depending on where they are located. To our knowledge no comparable programs are yet available in Nova Scotia, although the need for enhanced transition services into and out of LTC in Nova Scotia were recommended in the report submitted in 2018 by the Minister's Expert Advisory Panel on Long-Term Care.

It is clear that closing the gaps in the provision of optimum care in Nova Scotia long-term care facilities will take some time to address. It is of note that there will also always be a two-tiered system of care, where those who have the means to pay can access well-appointed, upscale residential care options while others will not have the required funds. The same will be true of options such as dementia villages where the development is being spearheaded by for-profit developers. This gap may only be closed when we figure out how to close the gap between the rich and the poor. Such villages should be public. That might help close the gap.

The Gap in Community Accessibility — Dementia-Friendly Communities

A dementia-friendly community provides community-based support and services through local action for those living with, or impacted by, dementia. A dementia-friendly community can be determined by both the social environment and the physical environment of the community. The Alzheimer's Society of the United Kingdom defines such a community this as "one in which people with dementia are empowered to have high aspirations and feel confident, knowing they can contribute and participate in activities that are meaningful to them" (Alzheimer's Society of the United Kingdom n.d.a).

In January of 2020, the Public Health Agency of Canada announced funding to the Alzheimer Society of Canada to

> collaborate with and build on the work already done by the Alzheimer Societies of British Columbia, Manitoba, Ontario and Saskatchewan to create the vision of dementia-friendly communities across Canada. A dementia-friendly community is a community where people living with dementia are understood, respected and supported. It is an environment where people are aware of and understand dementia and where people living with dementia are included and have a choice in and control over their day-to-day lives and level of engagement. (Government of Canada 2020)

To support a consistent approach across the country, the four provincial Alzheimer Societies will engage with both rural and urban centres. The Alzheimer Society of Canada will develop a national Dementia-Friendly Canada (DFC) toolkit, which will include guides and tools to educate and train professionals in a variety of areas, such as transportation, recreation, libraries and the service sector. It will also include a module for the general public. Knowledge exchange events will be held to help distribute the DFC toolkit, as well as any other developed resources. A national dementia-friendly website will also be created to showcase these new resources, as well as other relevant tools and related links (Government of Canada 2020).

The Government of Alberta has produced a very interesting and useful toolkit to assist communities who wish to establish a dementia-friendly atmosphere. It can be found at dementiafriendlyalberta.ca and is called *A Guide for Creating Dementia Friendly Communities in Alberta* (Alberta Health Services 2021). Similar initiatives exist in other Canadian provinces as well as internationally.

For example, in Scotland, dementia-friendly communities were first created in 2012, starting with the small town of Motherwell. The aim of such communities is to assist persons with dementia to get around the environment as easily as possible. The latest such community, Aberfeldy, is inviting the entire town to become involved. An October 31, 2019, article by Elizabeth Quigley on the BBC's website notes:

> From cafes and bookshops to the post office and the cinema, the whole community is involved.
>
> For instance, members of the Aberfeldy Rotary Club learned that a simple change of colour can make a world of difference.
>
> They are changing the white toilet seat in a disabled toilet in a cafe to a coloured one.
>
> This can help people differentiate the toilet seat from the bowl, which can be confusing and embarrassing. (Quigley 2019)

These towns and communities also provide awareness training for key staff in all local shops and services, such as banks, libraries, cafés and so on, and the town and village planners were also involved in looking at clear and concise signage, ease of navigation, lighting, seating areas and types of flooring.

These strategies for improving dementia care at all levels, including community-based design and planning, are in keeping with the suggestions of the Alzheimer Society of Canada and the Alzheimer's Disease International 2020 report, written by Professor Richard Fleming, Dr. John Zeisel and Kirsty Bennett and titled *Design, Dignity, Dementia: Dementia-Related Design and the Built Environment*. In this report, a group of eight international dementia researchers gathered together to discuss the need to do things differently in the construction of long-term care facilities for people with dementia. It was noted that design for people with dementia is thirty years behind that of the physical disabilities movement. It was agreed by all in the discussion groups how important the role of appropriate design was.

Dementia-friendly communities are one way to improve accessibility for persons living with dementia and the people who care for them. However, a more accessible community also helps all of us as our friends and nieghbours living with dementia can continue to live at home longer and this models to everyone the way in which the community values all its members.

The Gap in Getting a Diagnosis and Navigating the Dementia Care Options

Several of the caregivers we interviewed had trouble getting a diagnosis for the person for whom they were providing care. They indicated that it sometimes took months, if not years, to get a diagnosis, that then was often vague (cognitive decline versus dementia) and occasionally seemed totally off-target (late-onset ADHD). Once diagnosed, navigating the dementia care options could also be problematic. Options that looked promising were not be available across the province while other services had long waitlists, and people who eventually accessed funding were often not made aware that it was available.

Geriatric and Dementia Care Clinics

There are four geriatric and dementia care clinics in Nova Scotia. Two are located at the Veteran's Memorial wing of the Camp Hill Hospital in Halifax. The Geriatric Ambulatory Care/Memory Disability Clinic sees mostly seniors (people 65 and over) with health problems related to frailty or dementia. A request needs to be sent by a primary care provider as consultations are on a referral basis only. The Geriatrics/Centre for Health Care for the Elderly (CHCE) is also located in the same facility. Its website states that it is

> a multi-service, interdisciplinary program based primarily in the Camp Hill Veterans' Memorial Building (CHVMB) of the Queen Elizabeth II Health Sciences Centre, Central Zone, Nova Scotia Health Authority. The cornerstone of our care is interdisciplinary

comprehensive geriatric assessment, treatment and education of frail older persons and their families. There is a prominent role of research, centered in the Geriatric Medicine Research Unit. (Nova Scotia Health Authority n.d.b)Q

The mission statements of this organization are to

- assist this population's response to challenges of aging successfully;
- maintain/optimize their quality of life;
- optimize functional ability;
- enhance access to health services;
- promote discussion of goals of medical care and to facilitate appropriate ways of implementing this in practice using such tools as advanced directives;
- help maintain a safe environment to assist people to stay in their homes if they wish and to promote independent living where possible;
- educate and support family members/caregivers regarding the trajectory of the patient's illness, without compromising their own emotional and physical health;
- undertake teaching and research, in geriatrics and gerontology;
- promote the interest of elderly people in the distribution of health care and other resources;
- combat ageism and all forms of abuse of the elderly; and
- advocate and uphold respect for the elderly. (Nova Scotia Health Authority n.d.b)

The website does not say how these objectives are met, or by whom, or where the services are conducted, which makes attempting to track down services challenging.

In Dartmouth at the General Hospital there is a Geriatric Navigator — a community program that offers in-home health assessments to people living in Dartmouth who are frail and elderly (clients 65 years and older). According to the Nova Scotia Health Authority (n.d.a), the assessments can include

- cognitive testing;
- mood assessment;
- mobility assessment;

- functional assessments (meal preparation, personal care, shopping needs, medication compliance);
- home safety; and
- assessment of community supports.

Following the assessment, the geriatric navigator makes recommendations regarding community resources that may be helpful to allow people to remain in their homes and improve their quality of life. Also after the assessment, a written report is sent to the family doctor, and if necessary and approved, follow-up home visits are arranged based on the client's abilities and needs.

Another example of a facility which aims to assist persons with dementia and their important ones is located in Antigonish at St. Martha's Regional Hospital, Nursing, Geriatric Assessment Clinic.

Free memory tests are conducted through the True North Clinical Research group, which has two locations in Nova Scotia — one in New Minas in the Annapolis Valley and the other in Halifax for those living in HRM and beyond. The goals of this organization are to collect data to be used in clinical trails into research examining medications that may be useful in helping treat Alzheimer's disease and other dementias. Their website points out that persons who request a memory test are in no way obligated to participate in research. Their website notes the following:

True North Clinical Research provides free memory testing that allows individuals to gauge the current state of their memory. To accomplish this, we perform two tests, the MMSE (Mini Mental State Examination) and the FCSRT (Free and Cued Selective Reminding Test). The FCSRT is very sensitive at detecting subtler, mild memory loss that other assessments may not pick up on. The memory assessment appointment is approximately 30 minutes in length. Each participant has the option to have his or her results saved in our database and the option to be invited back for re-testing in the future. As Alzheimer's disease is a progressive impairment in memory, these options allow individuals and True North Clinical Research to track memory abilities over time. Individual's memory test scores can also be shared with each individual's family doctor. (True North Clinical Research n.d.)

Several of the caregivers with whom we spoke mentioned that their family member had attended the programs provided through True North's services for memory testing.

In email correspondence (received from Kristie Creighton, Manager, Program Developer on January 28, 2021) with the Alzheimer Society of Nova Scotia we were informed that

> there are about 36 NSH clinicians who are providing geriatric services/care throughout the province but unfortunately, there is no comprehensive list with # of memory clinics for the province. This info is from a research team looking at mapping dementia care in the province, led by Dr. Paula McLaughlin.

Dr. Paula McLaughlin and her colleagues at Nova Scotia Health have received funding from the QEII Foundation to investigate the current needs of persons with dementia and to identify ways to improve dementia care in the province.

Navigating the dementia care system can be challenging for people who have been newly diagnosed. The concept of a Community Geriatric Navigator as currently offered in Dartmouth would help people make connections with services sooner. Accessing services early on in the dementia journey has been shown to have positive effects on the quality of life for persons living with dementia and those who care for them.

The Gap in Respite Care Services

In the interviews with caregivers, one of the greatest challenges they highlighted was accessing respite care. This was particularly true during the pandemic, but caregivers stated that it is generally true of nighttime respite.

Day and Night Respite Programs

Adult day programs for older persons are provided throughout the province of Nova Scotia in a variety of settings, most providing programming that allows caregivers to drop off their loved ones with dementia for up to six hours a day. While present in the program, often located in community centres, hospitals or other community-based settings, they provide an opportunity for people to socialize, engage in activities intended to increase mobility and stamina, assist with preparing lunches, listen to guest speakers or watching videos. Adult day programs may be offered by private companies and organizations within a nursing home or residential care facility. There is a fee charged for these services. For a list of these programs, go to the Caregivers Nova Scotia website (Caregivers Nova Scotia n.d.).

All long-term care facilities in Nova Scotia provide respite care beds for patients and their families who need a short-term stay for a minimal cost. The website for Continuing Care in Nova Scotia provides the following information about this service:

> A respite bed gives a person who needs personal care a place to stay for a scheduled amount of time where he/she can continue to receive care and support from long-term care facility staff when his/her regular caregiver is unavailable. During his/her stay, the person gets the necessary care and support, including meals, from the facility staff, and returns home at the end of the scheduled time in the facility. (Province of Nova Scotia n.d.a)

To schedule a respite bed the following rules apply:

> You can apply for a respite bed by calling 1-800-225-7225 (toll free). A Care Coordinator will assess the applicant's care needs and eligibility. Once the applicant is confirmed eligible for the service, the Care Coordinator will arrange for a respite bed for the applicant on a first-come, first served basis. (Province of Nova Scotia n.d.a)

In Nova Scotia the provincial government does provide a caregiver benefit which recognizes the important role of caregivers in their efforts to assist loved ones and friends. The program is intended for caregivers of low-income adults who have a high level of disability or impairment, as determined by a Home Care assessment. If the caregiver and the care recipient both qualify for the program, the caregiver will receive $400 per month. In order to receive this benefit, the following eligibility requirements must be met. The care-receiver must

> have a net annual income of $22,125 or less if single, or a total net household income of $37,209 or less, if married or common-law. They must have been assessed by a Nova Scotia Health Authority care coordinator as having a high level of impairment or disability requiring significant care over time. (Province of Nova Scotia n.d.c)

To receive the benefit, both the caregiver and the person for whom they provide care must meet the program's eligibility criteria. The Nova Scotia Health Authority determines eligibility through a referral and assessment process. The Caregiver Benefit is reportable income so caregivers should contact the Canada Revenue Agency for information about tax implications.

If an individual is receiving support from the province's Continuing Care program, they may be eligible for the Continuing Supportive Care Grant. The Supportive Care Program supports eligible Nova Scotians with cognitive impairments (difficulty thinking, concentrating, remembering, etc.) by providing them with up to $1000 per month for Home Support Services (personal care, respite, meal preparation and household chores). Under this program people may also be eligible to receive reimbursement for snow removal services up to $495 per year. To receive funding for supportive care, you must

- Be 65 years of age or older (or be diagnosed with dementia or an acquired brain injury if under 65).
- Be a Nova Scotia resident with a valid Health Card.
- Have significant memory loss and memory problems that affect daily functioning.
- Be deemed by Continuing Care as needing a minimum of 25 hours/month of care support.
- Have a Substitute Decision Maker (someone who will act on your behalf and has signed an agreement that defines terms and conditions for this program). (Province of Nova Scotia n.d.c)

While private agencies can be used to supply these services, family members cannot be funded as noted below:

Funding under this program cannot be used to purchase services from:

- A person or organization providing home support and/or snow removal services and who also owns, rents or manages the household/facility the client lives in (e.g., an assisted living facility).
- Family members of a Supportive Care client, including a spouse/partner, children/ grandchildren, parent/grandparent, siblings, aunts/uncles and nephews/nieces. (Province of Nova Scotia n.d.c)

Other than those provided by private agencies, we could find no night respite services; however, in British Columbia the Health and Home Care Society of BC provides an overnight respite care program for families and other caregivers of persons with dementia, as well as other conditions. This program is offered seven days a week, every day of the year. The facility offers twelve private rooms with their own washrooms. It also provides a dedicated nursing team and assistance with personal care (Health and Home Care Society of BC 2020).

As well, Fraser Valley Health, which is one of five regional health authorities in BC, working together with the Ministry of Health, provides overnight respite care through the delivery of hospital and community-based health services.

In discussions with a friend whose father had received overnight respite care when he was experiencing COPD (chronic obstructive pulmonary disease) while living in the Annapolis Valley, Jeanette was told that the agency which provided this service charged $25 per hour per night, but that they required that the care provider be in the home for at least three nights a week. Although her father lived in Nova Scotia, she and her two siblings lived in another province on the West Coast so they could not care for him in his home.

One of the people we interviewed, John, had mentioned that he tried to find overnight care for his wife who is living with dementia. He also lives in the Annapolis Valley, and in a recent telephone call update John said that he was unable to find someone through a care agency as none were available, but he was able to find a retired nurse who does provide respite care in the daytime, as well as night, through a neighbour's church. He pays the care provider $30 an hour. He said that while his wife was comfortable with the care provider in the daytime, she was confused, agitated and frightened at night, so "it wasn't worth the risk of upsetting her further, so I just manage as best I can on my own."

To find out more about the accessibility and costs involved in receiving overnight respite care for the loved ones of persons with dementia, we conducted a very informal survey. We contacted six private home care agencies — three in HRM and the same number in the Annapolis Valley. While most were local companies, one was part of a major national chain. The average cost per hour for overnight respite care for persons with dementia was between $26.50 and $30 per hour. Two agencies said that they could not provide services for less than three nights. The others said it depended on the assessments which would be done prior to a contract being signed for services. In all cases they said that the services would be provided based on which stage of dementia the patient was living with, which would be determined at assessment, and if, in the opinion of the assessor, they could not handle that level of care, they could refuse to supply service. In all cases, those providing care would be CCAs (community care assistants). All but two agencies had staff available currently. The others said that they had waiting lists. While it is good to know that such public services exist, it is problematic that the costs are so high and that only those with higher incomes can benefit from them.

One of the changes in the life of caregivers that would have the greatest impact on them and those they care for would be access to nighttime respite care as a public service at an affordable price. It is this challenge that resulted in many caregivers having their family member assessed for long-term care. Closing this gap does not appear on the agenda of policy makers but it might be one of the most effective ways to slow up the demand for long-term care beds.

The Gap in Planning for Dementia Care

While the Baby Boom has affected demography in Canada (and much of the world) since it was first recognized following World War II and extending to the early 1960s, the required planning for late-life services does not appeared to have kept up. Alzheimer's societies have been putting out the warning for years, but for just as long Baby Boomers have thought of dementia as a condition that affects their grandparents or parents. As the Boomers enter their mid-seventies the time gap on planning is closing fast.

National and International Plans for Dealing with Dementia

Alzheimer's Disease International, located in the United Kingdom, provides a list of the thirty-seven countries and territories which have developed dementia plans as of January 2020. Twenty-nine of them are part of the WHO (World Health Organization) Initiatives member states. The organization notes that unlike international initiatives, national plans are capable of addressing dementia issues in a way that is tailored to the unique culture and demographics of each country. The WHO Global Plan on Dementia urges that all governments develop national policies on dementia by 2025:

A comprehensive government plan to address the needs of people with dementia can provide a mechanism to consider a range of issues including promoting public awareness of dementia and improving the quality of health care, social care and long-term care support and services for people living with dementia and their families. (Alzheimer's Disease International n.d.c)

The countries in the list, including the dates when their government policies were created, with definite plans are the following:

Australia — National Framework for Action on Dementia (2015–2019)
Austria — Dementia Strategy: Living Well with Dementia (2015)
Bulgaria — National Action Plan (2015)
Canada — A Dementia Strategy for Canada: Together We Aspire (2019)
Chile — Plan Nacional de Demencia (2017–2025)
Costa Rica — National Plan (2014–2024)
Cuba — Strategy for Alzheimer Disease and Dementia Syndromes (2016)
Czech Republic — National Plan (2016–2019)
Denmark — Dementia Action Plan (2017–2025)
Finland — National Memory Plan (2012–2020)
France — Plan maladies neuro-dégénératives (2014–2019)
Greece — National Dementia Strategy (2016–2020)
Indonesia — National Dementia Strategy (2016)
Ireland — National Dementia Strategy (2011–2016)
Israel — National Program for Addressing Alzheimer's Disease and Other Types of Dementia (2013)
Italy — National Dementia Strategy (2014)
Japan — Orange Plan (2015)
Korea, Republic of — National Dementia Plan (2015)
Luxembourg — National Dementia Action Plan (2013)
Malta — Empowering Change (2015–2023)
Mexico — Plan de Accion Alzheimer Y otras Demencias (2014)
Netherlands — National Dementia Program (2012–2020)
Norway — Dementia Plan (2015–2020)
Qatar — National Dementia Plan (2018–2022 Summary)
Singapore — National Dementia Strategy (2009)
Slovenia — National Plan (2016–2020)

Spain — National Health System Strategy for Neurodegenerative Diseases (2016)
Switzerland — National Dementia Strategy (2014–2019)
USA — National Alzheimer's Plan (2017: 2018 Update)

Countries with government plans in development or being changed are Belgium, Germany, Switzerland, England, Northern Ireland, Wales, Scotland, Gibraltar, Puerto Rico, Macau, Chinese Taipei and New Zealand (Alzheimer's Disease International n.d.b).

For more information on theses specific dementia plans, we suggest that you go to the website of Alzheimer's Disease International at alzint.org. Noticeably absent from these plans are countries in the continent of Africa, as well as those in South America and the Middle East. Most of these plans, including Canada's, are based on guidelines produced by the World Health Organization in their 2017 report, *Global Action Plan on the Public Health Response to Dementia 2017–2025*. The report was produced after ten years of advocacy for a global response to dementia by Alzheimer's Disease International and other organizations worldwide.

The goal of the plan aims to "improve the lives of people with dementia, their families and the people who care for them, while decreasing the impact of dementia on communities and countries. It provides a comprehensive blueprint for action and sets targets across seven areas" (Alzheimer's Disease International n.d.c).

The six areas identified in the plan produced by the WHO (2017) are:

- dementia as a public health priority;
- dementia awareness and friendliness;
- dementia risk reduction;
- dementia diagnosis;
- treatment, care and support; and
- information systems for dementia and dementia research and innovation.

The Canadian Plan

The Canadian Action Plan for Dementia (*A Dementia Strategy for Canada: Together We Aspire*) is based on five principles:

- Collaboration — Achieving progress on the strategy is a shared responsibility among governments, researchers, community organizations, people living with dementia, caregivers and many others.

- Research and innovation — Promoting research and innovation will address knowledge gaps and develop therapies that will improve the quality of life of people with dementia and caregivers and move us towards a cure.
- Surveillance and data — Enhanced surveillance and data will help us to understand the scope of dementia in Canada and focus our efforts and resources where they are most needed and will be most effective.
- Information resources — The development of culturally appropriate and culturally safe information resources on dementia will facilitate the work of care providers to provide quality care and will help all Canadians to better understand dementia.
- Skilled workforce — Having a sufficient and skilled workforce will support dementia research efforts and provide evidence-informed care, which will improve the quality of life of people living with dementia and caregivers. (Government of Canada 2019)

Based on these principles the following three objectives were identified:

1. Prevent dementia
2. Advance therapies and find a cure
3. Improve the quality of life of people living with dementia and caregivers. (Government of Canada 2019)

The strategy is intended to place emphasis on those groups who are at a higher risk of dementia as well as those who face barriers to equitable care:

These groups include but are not limited to Indigenous peoples, individuals with intellectual disabilities, individuals with existing health issues such as hypertension and Type 2 diabetes, older adults, women, ethnic and cultural minority communities, LGBTQ2 individuals, official language minority communities, rural and remote communities and those with young onset dementia. (Government of Canada 2019)

According to the Alzheimer Society of Canada, in 2019, the year that the Government of Canada released its federal dementia plan, five provinces had strategies or dementia action plans in place or are in the process of developing their own dementia strategies: Nova Scotia, Quebec (French only), Ontario, Alberta and British Columbia. In addition, some provinces and territories, such as New Brunswick, are developing seniors' strategies that will address dementia as well. (Alzheimer Society of Canada n.d.c)

The Nova Scotia Plan, titled *Towards Understanding: A Dementia Strategy for Nova Scotia,* was produced in June 2015 and follows many of the same guidelines as those in the federal plan. To reach the objectives the province will develop an action strategy and plan; gather insight and input from geriatric specialists and organizations providing support to persons with dementia and their caregivers; utilize a person-centred approach because as the authors suggest, "Experiencing dementia is a personal journey which differs for each individual and their family/caregiver. It is critical that health care providers and the health system generally takes into account this personal journey when interacting with individuals, their families and caregivers" (Nova Scotia Department of Health and Wellness. 2015: 6). The next strategy identified in the plan is to create a Framework for Action, then to measure the plan's "Reality, Response, Results" (Nova Scotia Department of Health and Wellness 2015: 9). At the time of writing, we were unable to find an update on this plan, or what steps have been taken to achieve the stated objectives.

The development of dementia plans or strategies by countries or provinces sets objectives to help guide actions by all levels of government, non-governmental organizations, communities, families and individuals. In the coming years with the increased number of people projected to be living with dementia, it will also provide a way to hold each other accountable to keep this challenge in the public eye and to live up to commitments.

The Gap in Memory Supports for Persons with Dementia

It seemed that every caregiver we interviewed had established ways to support the memory of the person for whom they were caring: memory books to Post-it notes, recorded messages to logbooks and iPad caregivers. In addition to these standard approaches, companies and products have been developed for just this purpose.

In the online publication produced by Age Watch in the United

Kingdom, a variety of such aids are listed. The website note:

> As we get older, we may find ourselves forgetting things more
> often. People living with dementia, and their carers, know bet-
> ter than anyone how distressing this can be. However, there are
> several new technologies to help people with dementia retain
> their independence, enabling them to continue to live at home
> for as long as possible. Many of these technologies are fairly new
> and include "assistive technologies" such as virtual assistants,
> electronic reminders and tracking devices. (Age Watch n.d.)

The article by Age Watch (n.d.) introduces some of the newer, but
widely available, technologies such as "virtual assistants," but it also
includes more traditional technologies such as specially adapted phones
and medication aids:

- "assistive" technologies
- "virtual assistants"
- automatic calendar clocks
- dementia-friendly phones
- GPS tracking
- assistive technologies for carers

What's next for assistive technology?

- robot pets
- medication aids
- reminder messages
- reminiscence and leisure aids
- safety aids
- AT memory aids
- recommendations and considerations.

For more information about each of these assistive technology devices
and descriptions of them go to the Age Watch website. While many of
these assistive devices are available in the United Kingdom and can be
rented for free from the Alzheimer's Society United Against Dementia
(located in the UK) and some of its subsidiaries, not all are available in
Canada. Age Watch (n.d.) recommends that loved ones of persons with
dementia consider the following when choosing or using memory aids:

1. Aids which may work for one person with dementia may not work for another. Remember to keep the use of aids person-centred. Tailor them to the needs and interests of the specific person with dementia rather than taking a one-size-fits-all approach.
2. Involve the person with dementia in the decisions about which memory aids to use.
3. Use technological aids to complement good care.
4. Memory aids which can be easily integrated into the routine of the person with dementia will cause least disruption and therefore may work best.
5. Start using memory aids as early as possible as they work best during the early stages of dementia.
6. Some people with dementia may prefer not to use memory aids, as they may view them as constant reminders of their memory problems. Where possible, only use memory aids with the consent of the person with dementia.

The nursing home complex where Jeanette is on the board has recently purchased a Mobii device to encourage interaction and engagement with persons with dementia (the first facility in the Annapolis Valley to do so). The device is an interactive floor/table one. It is a fully portable projection system with one-button height adjustment; it can be taken wherever needed and projects onto bedsides, dining tables, floors and walls, making it interactive and intergenerational for when family comes to visit, especially younger people. The Mobii includes a variety of programs and tasks for residents to complete, encouraging and assisting with movement and mobility, creativity and stretching. The unit is a therapeutic tool for engagement in activities; it includes music and very colourful images to further inspire. For a very interesting video on the ways in which this system can be used, especially in nursing homes and other long-term care facilities, go to the OM Interactive website (OM Interactive n.d.).

Staff at the facility report that residents with dementia are highly motivated and amused by the device and much laughter is heard down the hallways when the Mobii is being used.

Memory aids appear to be limited only by one's imagination and the ability to access the aid. The gap that may need to be closed is the cost of the aids.

The Gap in Medical Assistance in Dying

Some of the caregivers we interviewed discussed the topic of Medical Assistance in Dying (MAID) and spoke about the ways in which, prior to a dementia diagnoses, their loved ones told them that in the event that they could no longer consent to MAID due to a medical condition, they would wish to have it. Because at that time it was not available to persons with dementia or other mental health symptoms, this was not possible. However, with the new legislation (Bill C-7) proposed by the federal government having received approval from the Senate and royal assent as of March 17, 2021, persons with dementia may apply for this assistance (Bryden 2021).

At the request of members of the Senate,

> The Government of Canada recognizes that other important outstanding issues related to MAID must still be explored. Areas such as the eligibility of mature minors, advance requests, mental illness, palliative care and the protection of Canadians living with disabilities will be considered during a parliamentary review of the MAID legislation that would begin within the next 30 days. (Department of Justice Canada 2021)

Prior to the new legislation being approved, Dr. Jocelyn Downie, a professor of Law and Medicine at Dalhousie University in Halifax, Nova Scotia, noted in October 2020:

> On October 5, 2020, the federal Minister of Justice introduced Bill C-7 to amend Canada's medical assistance in dying (MAID) legislation. Parliament will debate this bill over the coming weeks, aiming to bring the legislation into force by December 18. One critical question about this bill for hundreds of thousands of Canadians is its implications for people with dementia (most commonly caused by Alzheimer's disease). The short answer is that more people with dementia will have access to MAID, since the legislation allows an advance request for the service before the loss of decision-making capacity. (Downie 2020)

Dr. Downie notes further that nothing in Bill C-7 changes the fact that some people with dementia (who still have decision-making capacity) will be legally permitted to receive MAID. According to Downie (2020), under the current and new law, a person can receive MAID if

- they have a serious and incurable illness, disease, or disability;
- they are in an advanced state of irreversible decline in capability;
- the illness, disease, or disability or the state of decline causes them enduring physical or psychological suffering that is intolerable to them and cannot be relieved under conditions that they consider acceptable; and
- their natural death has become reasonably foreseeable, taking into account all of their medical circumstances, without a prognosis necessarily having been made as to the specific length of time that they have remaining.

People with dementia (even as their sole underlying medical condition) can meet these criteria. Dementia is a serious and incurable illness, disease or disability ("major neurocognitive disorder"). A person with dementia can be in an advanced state of irreversible decline in capability before losing decision-making capacity (Downie 2020).

While for some this topic is a contentious one, for persons with dementia and their loved ones who wish for this medical procedure to be provided when they choose it, this is important news and has closed the gap for those living with dementia who wish to exercise this option.

The Gap in Understanding Dementia as Addressed in the Arts and Social Media

The arts have the potential for transformative power for those who are participants and those who are observers. Creative pursuits can both transform individual lives and create social change. For this reason, it is important to support bridging the understanding gap by encouraging people with dementia to participate in artistic pursuits and encouraging artists of all sorts to share information about dementia.

For twenty years or more, movies have been made and books written on the topic of dementia, many receiving critical acclaim. Here are some of them:

- *The Father* (Movie — starring Sir Anthony Hopkins, who was nominated for a Golden Globe for his performance and won an Oscar, 2020)

- *Elizabeth Is Missing* (Movie — Starring Glenda Jackson, 2019; Book — Emma Healy, 2014)
- *What They Had* (Movie — starring Hilary Swank and Michael Shannon, 2018)
- *Still Alice* (Movie — Starring Julianne Moore, who won an Oscar for her performance, 2015; Book — Lisa Genova, 2007)
- *Mr. Holmes* (Movie — starring Sir Ian McKellan, 2014)
- *The Iron Lady* (Movie — starring Meryl Streep, for which she won a Golden Globe Award among others, 2012)
- *The Savages* (Movie — starring Laura Linney and Philip Seymour Hoffman, 2008)
- *Away From Her* (Movie — starring Julie Christie and Gordon Pinsent, 2007; Book — from a short story collection written by Alice Munro, 2007).
- *The Notebook* (Movie — Starring Ryan Gosling and Rachel McAdams, 2004; Book — Nicholas Sparks, 1996)
- *Iris: A Memoir of Iris Murdoch* (Movie — Starring Judi Dench as the older Iris and Kate Winslet as the younger, 2002; Book — John Bayley, her husband, 1998)

While the majority of these movies and books feature dementia in the lives of women, *The Father* and *Mr. Holmes* have male lead characters, reinforcing to the public that dementia is experienced by all sexes. What all these movies have in common is that they provide glimpses into the lives of individuals and families dealing with the subject of dementia and Alzheimer's disease.

In addition, novels such as *And Every Morning the Way Home Gets Longer* (Fredrik Backman, 2016), *A Sudden Light* (Garth Stein, 2014), *We Are Not Ourselves* (Matthew Thomas, 2014), *Turn of Mind* (Alice LaPlante, 2011) and *Memory Board* (Jane Rule, 1987) among others provide another look into the fictional but realistic experiences of persons living with dementia and being given care for it. For a more complete list of the novels written on this topic, goodreads.com is a good source.

Another component of media which addresses dementia is that of books written for children. A social worker in Britsh Columbia named Olivia provides a list of some of these titles on her website, thiswestcoast-mommy.com, in a blog called "12 Children's Books to Help Your Child Understand Dementia and Alzheimer's" (West Coast Mommy n.d.).

Alzheimers Net also provides a list of titles written specifically for young readers in an article called "Books for Children About Alzheimer's and Dementia" (Alzheimers.net. n.d.). Similarly, the Alzheimer's Society of the United Kingdom has a list of recommended books entitled "Recommended Books about Dementia for Children and Teenagers" (Alzheimer's Society of the United Kingdom n.d.b).

As well as movies and books, music and songs in all genres, such as country, pop, rock and hip-hop, also deal with dementia. Some examples are listed in an article by Joe Oliveto on March 3, 2021, titled "15 Famous Songs about Dementia or Alzheimer's" (Oliveto 2021).

All of these popular sources of entertainment bring the topic of dementia into the awareness of the public and in that way provide a focus on the topic which in turn prompts awareness, discussion and increased understanding.

In a very interesting article titled "Forgotten but Not Gone: Dementia in the Arts" in the British newspaper *The Guardian*, author Philip Ball discusses various projects based in the arts that help persons with dementia express themselves through art therapy projects. He references a program called Created Out of Mind. Here is a description from their website:

> Launched in October 2016, and working over a period of 22 months, Created Out of Mind are the second residents of The Hub — a unique, creative space at Wellcome Collection in London. Starting with people with dementias, Created Out of Mind is an interdisciplinary team of scientists, visual artists, musicians, broadcasters, clinicians and carers. (Created Out of Mind n.d.)

Created Out of Mind is the brainchild of Sebastian Crutch, a neuropsychologist at the Dementia Research Centre of University College London. As well as challenging stereotypes about what it means to live with dementia, the project aims to

> develop better tools for assessing the value of using arts with people who have these conditions. All too often, such efforts are perceived as "giving them something to do," or perhaps as utilitarian therapies for sustaining cognitive skills. But if the real personal enrichment of the arts often comes "in the moment," why should it be any different for people with dementia? And

such activities can reveal a creativity obscured by impairment of an individual's resources for regular communication. (Ball 2017)

As well as art projects such as drawing and illustrations, the program also offers poetry writing workshops, movie making, music making, self-portraits, singing, pottery and ceramic making and many other forms of artistic expression. Crutch notes:

> Dementia is mostly, and rightly, associated with deficits of one kind or another in mental abilities. But the mind is extraordinarily inventive about circumventing difficulties or improvising with what it has to hand, and it's not so surprising then that these neural gymnastics might introduce new aspects of personality, new interests and capacities. These might be puzzling or bewildering to people who see a loved one change, but as Harvey attests, the results need not be solely negative. Someone might develop a hitherto unseen passion for opera. They might take up painting with almost manic energy. Or they might discover new facets of their creativity. (Ball 2017)

Another project based in the United Kingdom is called Living Words. This is a charitable organization which encourages and supports persons with dementia to express themselves through the written word in the form of poetry and other literary projects. According to their website, the program

> enable[s] participants' experience in the moment to be heard by others: at the end of our projects, participants have their own book of their "Living Words" that express how they feel about life; and we run staff workshops to support creative expression and embed use of the Living Words books.
>
> Our writers also work in an ongoing fashion with privately funded individuals, often over many years. Inspired by all this participatory work we create anthologies, performances, films, artworks, songs, podcasts and events.
>
> We believe that if a person is believed in, valued and given a non-judgmental space in which to express themselves, everyone benefits.
>
> We have continued guidance from our team of individuals

living with dementia, as well as senior professionals within the field of dementia care and research. (Living Words n.d.)

A number of communities (including some in Canada) have started dementia choirs. One such choir started in Victoria in 2018, and is called Voices in Motion. The choir included people living with dementia, their caregivers and high school students. The high school students were brought into the choir in an attempt to start reducing the societal stigma around dementia, one connection at a time. In an article by *The Tyee*, the choir organizers note

> The project has grown to three choirs, indicating that we need more such programs that celebrate the potential of living well with dementia, as well as helping society itself become more dementia-friendly. Studies show that the choral experience helps singers with dementia recall details from long-buried memories, increases functioning memory, decreases distress among caregivers and reduces stigma while increasing empathy across age groups. These are verifiable, non-pharmaceutical benefits. (Sheets et al. 2020)

When COVID-19 hit, the choirs went online and an online community blossomed. Besides singing, people began sharing stories and experiences. The participants agree that the pandemic "helps us see that all levels of government need to support innovative ways to connect those with dementia to others, in person and online. Let's start with music as the universal, joyful operating system" (Sheets et al. 2020).

In the end it is possible that the gap in understanding dementia which results in fear and stigma may best be addressed through creative endeavours.

7

Losing Me

We all lose parts of ourselves when a loved one dies and our identity is entwined with theirs, but perhaps because their physical presence is gone it may be easier to deal with that loss. It is so much harder when that person is still sitting across from you at the kitchen table but doesn't acknowledge or recognize you or the roles you have played in their lives. We see ourselves reflected in the eyes and experiences of others and those realities shape our images of self and our presentation of self — as someone else's partner, lover, friend, parent, sibling, neighbour and so on. When we are no longer visible to important ones due to dementia, who are we as we look in the mirror and how does it feel to see them (or who they used to be) disappear before us? This was one of the topics we wanted to explore in our conservations with caregivers.

We found that caregivers spoke about losing themselves as they were losing their loved ones in the following ways:

Lost relationship — caregivers moving from connectedness to loneliness as the dementia progresses is one of the ways in which they feel that they were starting to lose their own identity.

- Marion remembers being very frustrated, bossy and impatient at times with her husband Dick. She also missed their joint activities and felt really lonely as her partner disappeared before her very eyes.
- Shirley cared for her husband Bill as they journeyed through their dementia experiences. She said that while in the nursing home her husband's condition deteriorated and he "hardly knew who I was most days. It really changes your perception of who you are — or used to be. I suppose that makes more sense."

Fear and uncertainty — where caregivers know the end result of dementia but have no idea the path that will be taken to get there. This sense of powerlessness can erode the caregiver's confidence and sense of autonomy.

- Reg said that while caring for his wife, Nell, his feelings about himself have changed so that "I was afraid sometimes of what would happen to Nell if something happened to me. I probably drink more than I should too. Instead of a beer on the weekend, now I sometimes have one or two in the week, just to take the edge off, you know."
- While caring for his mother, Stella, Jeff was constantly changing his roles based on whether or not she remembered who he was. He said, "When I wake up in the mornings I often think 'Who will I be today?' I always wanted to be an actor, but not on this stage. There's just so many roles I could play in her mind, so I don't always know who I am either. It's a bit schizophrenic."
- Verline quipped, "My brother sometimes asks me, 'What's your plan?' I answer, 'Survival and it is not going to get any better.'"
- When asked if the experience of living with dementia has affected how she feels about herself, Jan said, "Definitely. I used to be a highly competent and confident woman, very politically astute and aware and an intellectual. Now I feel scared and anxious about what else I might lose as a result of this and just not myself anymore. It is not a good feeling and no matter how I try I cannot shake it off."

The role of caregiver predominates — in this case the caregiver feels the role subsumes all other roles and their identity is defined by this responsibility. We cited a friend of Jeanette's earlier in the book when she said,

We have been married for forty-two years. I was his wife, lover and best friend, mother of his children and confidant. I was also his memory keeper. Now he doesn't know who I am, and it is like I have been erased from his life, and mine. So, I don't know who I am anymore either.

Another friend said,

She has really bad memory lapses now, so sometimes she calls me Bob, who was her youngest brother. He has been dead for years. Some days I am not sure who I am. I am so tired that pretending

to be Bob is easier to deal with rather than reminding her that it's me, her husband of all these years.

Jane cared for her mother, Joyce, and recalls that in their family her mother looked after her mother (Jane's grandmother) and as a result she "changed. I am also changing. I am existing but I am losing myself."

Some of the caregivers suggested that their life was now a "roller coaster." When one rides a roller coaster, in addition to the excitement one feels there is a sense of fear and suspense as you wait to see what comes next — a feeling that "your stomach is in a blender" and a sense of powerlessness and surrendering to the ride. All relationships change over time but when one is caregiver to a person living with dementia it is possible to see how the constant and unpredictable changes might make one feel that their life was a roller coaster.

Some of the anxiety and stress that come from lost relationships, fear, uncertainty and being subsumed by caregiving responsibilities is the result of ambiguous loss. One type of ambiguous loss is defined as "a type of loss you feel when a person with dementia is physically here but may not be mentally or emotionally present in the same way as before." (Long, Favaro and Mulder 2017). The uncertainty of this loss can prevent people from adjusting to it, but it is possible to implement strategies to revise and broaden one's self-identity and thereby lower stress and reduce role confusion.

The Alzheimer Society of Canada has an excellent booklet addressing these experiences under the title "Ambiguous Loss and Grief in Dementia" (Alzheimer Society of Canada 2019c).

One's identity is influenced by multiple factors, including race, sexual orientation, cultural community, education, employment, interests, values and family. Identity changes over time to keep pace with the changes that happen in our lives. Changes like a new job, the death of a family member, a move, the end of a relationship, completion of a new level of training or education or becoming a parent result in others seeing us differently and us seeing ourselves in new ways as well. Persons may feel that they are losing themselves while providing care to an individual living with dementia because this person who is so important to them no longer sees them for who they are. Many caregivers are doing so as an extension of a pre-existing relationship (partner, daughter, friend for example), and when this connection is not recognized it can be devastating. In addition, caregiving can by its nature become isolating, and this puts the caregiver in a situation where they don't see people who can nurture other aspects of their self-identity. As a result, it is not surprising that some caregivers to persons living with dementia feel as though they are disappearing as the memory of their important one disappears.

Some caregivers have taken a step back from the label of "caregiver" saying instead that they are persons who provide care. They do this to make their personhood the primary focus. This change of language attempts to suggest that providing care is one aspect of who they are. The fact is that changes in language alone will not be enough.

It is important in the coming years to ensure that there are sufficient policies and programs in place to prevent caregivers of persons living with dementia from getting "lost" in their role. The caregivers who shared their stories have told us clearly what needs to change to prevent this role from becoming all consuming. Organizations and governments are starting to address these concerns (prompted in part by COVID-19) but it will take a groundswell of support from the community to ensure that the momentum for change continues.

Rosalynn Carter, the former first lady and wife of former president Jimmy Carter, has dedicated years to advocating for the needs of care-givers. She gives us a compelling reason to improve the lot of those who assume this role: "There are only four kinds of people in the world. Those who have been caregivers. Those who are currently caregivers. Those who will be caregivers, and those who will need a caregiver" (Rosalynn Carter Institute for Caregivers 2020: 4).

Appendix A

Questionnaire

1. What is your name? Age? Gender? Occupation? Race? Relationship to the subject?
   a. If the relationship is partner:
      i. How long were they married or living together?
      ii. Do they (either one of them) have children? If yes, where do the children live?
      iii. Is there other family close by?
   b. If the relationship is child:
      i. Where do you live?
      ii. How often do you interact with the subject?
      iii. How do you interact? (in person, by phone etc.)
   c. If the relationship is friend:
      i. How long have you known one another?
      ii. How often do you interact? (in person, by phone etc.)
2. What is the name of the subject? Age? Gender? Occupation? Race?
3. Tell me when you first noticed changes in the subject. What did you do about it? How did it make you feel?
4. When was the subject diagnosed with dementia? How old was the subject at the time of diagnosis?
5. What roles did the subject play in your life? (For example, beyond being husband was he primary earner, travel companion, etc.)
6. What roles did you play in the life of the subject (For example, beyond being wife were you family connector, household organizer, etc.)
7. What other roles did (do) you play in your family and/or community?
8. Did the subject's role(s) change as the dementia progressed? If yes, in what way?

9. Did your role(s) change as the dementia progressed? If yes, in what way?

10. Do you (or did you) receive any respite or support in your new role(s)? If so, from whom? Was there a cost for this service? Was the respite care adequate in terms of the quality or quantity of the care? If no, how did this affect you?

11. Did you ever feel overworked, time-stressed or burned out by your new role(s)?

12. Have you had someone you can count on to help you to make decisions as the dementia progressed?

13. Have the changing roles impacted your life? If yes, in what way?

14. Has your income been affected be the changing roles? If yes, how?

15. Has your community, friends or family responded to the subject's dementia and your new role(s)? If yes, describe.

16. Have you learned anything about yourself as a result of this experience? If yes, please explain.

17. Have there been any perceptible benefits to your new role(s)? If yes, what are they?

18. Has your faith contributed in any way to this experience? If yes, can you explain?

19. What coping strategies helped (or are helping) you to navigate the challenges presented by dementia?

20. Has this whole experience affected how you feel about yourself? If yes, in what way?

21. What recommendations would you make to others just starting the journey of caring for, or supporting someone with dementia?

22. Are there other aspects of this story you would like to expand on or share?

Bibliography

Age Watch. n.d. "Memory Aids for Dementia." <agewatch.net/mind/memory-aids-for-people-with-de/>.

Alberta Health Services. 2021. "A Guide for Creating Dementia Friendly Communities in Alberta." The Government of Alberta. <https://www.dementiafriendlyalberta.ca/>.

Alzheimer's Disease International. n.d.a "Alois Alzheimer." <alzint.org/about/dementia-facts-figures/types-of-dementia/alzheimers-disease/alois-alzheimer/>.

———. n.d.b. "Dementia Plans." <alzint.org/what-we-do/policy/dementia-plans/>.

———. n.d.c. "WHO Global Plan on Dementia." <alzint.org/what-we-do/partnerships/world-health-organization/who-global-plan-on-dementia/>.

Alzheimers.net. n.d. "Books for Children about Alzheimer's and Dementia." <alzheimers.net/6-03-16-books-for-children-about-alzheimers-and-dementia>.

Alzheimer Society of Canada. n.d.a. "Communication." Day to Day Series. <alzheimer.ca/sites/default/files/documents/day-to-day-series_communication.pdf>.

———. n.d.b. "How Your Intimate Relationships Can Change." <alzheimer.ca/en/help-support/im-living-dementia/managing-changes-your-abilities/how-your-intimate-relationships-can>.

———. n.d.c. "Canada's National Dementia Strategy." <alzheimer.ca/en/take-action/change-minds/canadas-national-dementia-strategy>.

———. n.d.d. "What Does Stigma Against Dementia Look Like?" <alzheimer.ca/en/about-dementia/stigma-against-dementia/what-does-stigma-against-dementia-look>.

———. n.d.e. "Managing Ambiguous Loss and Grief." <alzheimer.ca/en/help-support/i-have-friend-or-family-member-who-lives-dementia/managing-ambiguous-loss-grief>.

———. n.d.f. "The COVID-19 and Dementia Task Force." <https://alzheimer.ca/en/help-support/dementia-resources/managing-through-covid-19/covid-19-dementia-task-force>.

———. 2016. *First Link … your first step to living well with dementia.* <https://alzheimer.ca/sites/default/files/documents/asc_first_link_e.pdf>.

———. 2019a. "Other Types of Dementia." <alzheimer.ca/en/about-dementia/other-types-dementia>.

———. 2019b. "Limbic-Predominant Aged-Related TDP-43 Encephalopathy (LATE-NC) — a Newly Identified Form of Dementia." <archive.alzheimer.ca/sites/default/files/files/national/position-statements/late-nc_may-2019_en.pdf>.

____. 2019c. "Ambiguous Loss and Grief in Dementia." <https://archive.alzheimer.ca/sites/default/files/files/national/core-lit-brochures/ambiguous-loss-and-grief_for-individuals-and-families.pdf>.

____. 2020. "Race and Dementia." <alzheimer.ca/en/take-action/change-minds/race-dementia>.

Alzheimer Society of Nova Scotia. 2020. "Dementia and People of African Descent." <alzheimer.ca/ns/sites/ns/files/documents/updated%20Rack%20Card_HAAC_Sept%202020%5B1%5D.pdf>.

Alzheimer's Society of the United Kingdom. n.d.a. "Cultural Sensitivity and Awareness." <alzheimers.org.uk/dementia-professionals/dementia-experience-toolkit/how-recruit-people-dementia/cultural-sensitivity-and-awareness>.

____. n.d.b. "Recommended Books about Dementia for Children and Teenagers." <alzheimers.org.uk/recommended-books-about-dementia-children-and-teenagers>.

Assal, Frederic. 2019. "History of Dementia." *Journal of Frontal Neurological Science*, 44: 118–126 (April 30). doi: 10.1159/000494959.

Ball, Phillip. 2017. "Forgetting but Not Gone: Dementia and the Arts." *The Guardian*, March 11. <theguardian.com/science/2017/mar/11/forgetting-but-not-gone-dementia-and-the-arts-research-project-alzheimers>.

Battams, Nathan. 2017a. *A Snapshot of Family Work and Caregiving in Canada.* Vanier Institute of the Family. <precisely.ca/change/wp-content/uploads/2016/05/Vanier_2017-02-21_Snapshot_Caregiving-Work.pdf>.

____. 2017b. *Sharing a Roof: MultiGenerational Homes in Canada (2016 Census Update).* Vanier Institute of the Family. <https://vanierinstitute.ca/sharing-a-roof-multi-generational-homes-in-canada-2016-census-update/>.

Bewick, Teagan. 2016. "Nurses Can Make a Difference: Caring for Those Living with Dementia." *Australian Journal of Dementia Care.* <journalofdementiacare.com/nurses-can-make-a-difference-caring-for-those-living-with-dementia/>.

Bloomberg Business News. 2019. "Chinese Alzheimer's Drug to Launch Global Trials Amid Skepticism." December 29. <bloomberg.com/news/articles/2019-12-29/chinese-alzheimer-s-drug-to-launch-global-trials-amid-skepticism>.

Bowden, Olivia. 2020. "Culturally Relevant Dementia Care System's Missing Piece, Advocates Say." CBC *News.* Aug. 25.<cbc.ca/news/canada/ottawa/dementia-seniors-immigrants-programming-1.5697664>.

Bryden, Joan. 2021. "Senate Passes Bill C-7 to Expand Access to Medical Assistance in Dying." CBC *News.* March 17. <cbc.ca/news/politics/senate-passes-medical-assistance-dying-billc7-1.5954281>.

CADTH (Canadian Agency for Drugs and Technologies in Health). 2019. *Dementia Villages: Innovative Residential Care for People with Dementia.* <https://cadth.ca/dementia-villages-innovative-residential-care-people-dementia>.

Health and Home Care Society of BC. 2020. "Overnight Respite Program." <carebc.ca/overnight-respite-program.html>.

Caregivers Nova Scotia. n.d. "Capital Region." <caregiversns.org/resources/adult-day-programs/capital-region/>.

____. 2018. "The Caregivers Handbook (2018) — Updated Edition." <https://

caregiversns.org/resources/handbook/>.

Caring.com Staff. n.d. "Walks with a Shuffle." <caring.com/symptoms/alzheimers-symptoms/walks-with-a-shuffle>.

Cohen, Carole. 2008. "Consumer Fraud and Dementia — Lessons Learned from Conmen." *Dementia*, 7, 3: 283–285. <journals.sagepub.com/doi/pdf/10.1177/1471301208093284>.

Created Out of Mind. n.d. "Created Out of Mind: Shaping Perceptions of Dementias." <createdoutofmind.org>.

Curry, Paul. 2015. *Broken Homes: Nurses Speak Out on the State of Long-Term Care in Nova Scotia and Chart a Course for a Sustainable Future.* Nova Scotia Nurses' Union. <nsnu.ca/sites/default/files/Broken%20Homes%20Report%20Full.pdf>.

Dementia UK. n.d. "What Is Dementia?" <dementiauk.org/understanding-dementia/what-is-dementia/>.

Department of Justice Canada. 2021. "New Medical Assistance in Dying Legislation Becomes Law." *Cision.* <newswire.ca/news-releases/new-medical-assistance-in-dying-legislation-becomes-law-852933756.html>.

Downie, Jocelyn. 2020. "Medical Assistance in Dying Bill an Important Step Forward for Canadians with Dementia." *Policy Options Politiques.* <policyoptions.irpp.org/magazines/october-2020/medical-assistance-in-dying-bill-an-important-step-forward-for-canadians-with-dementia/>.

Fagen, Zara. 2013. "Chinese Herbs for Treating Alzheimers." Science of Natural Health. March 2. < scienceofnaturalhealth.com/treating-alzheimers.html>.

Fleming, R., J. Zeisel, and K. Bennett. 2020. *World Alzheimer Report 2020: Design, Dignity, Dementia: Dementia-Related Design and the Built Environment, Volume 1.* Alzheimer's Disease International and Alzheimer Society of Canada. <alzint.org/u/WorldAlzheimerReport2020Vol1.pdf>.

Frank, Christopher. 2018. "SMILE — Helping Dementia Caregivers." *Canadian Family Physician.* <cfp.ca/news/2018/03/06/03-05>.

Goodman, Brenda. 2019. "New Alzheimer's Drug from China: Hope or Hype?" WebMD. November 5. <webmd.com/alzheimers/news/20191105/new-alzheimers-drug-from-china-hope-or-hype>.

Government of Canada. 2018. *Framework on Palliative Care in Canada.* December 4. <https://www.canada.ca/en/health-canada/services/health-care-system/reports-publications/palliative-care/framework-palliative-care-canada.html>.

___. 2019. *A Dementia Strategy for Canada: Together We Aspire.* Public Health Agency, June. <canada.ca/en/public-health/services/publications/diseases-conditions/dementia-strategy.html>.

___. 2020. *Dementia Community Investment.* Public Health Agency of Canada. <canada.ca/en/public-health/news/2020/01/backgrounder-dementia-community-investment.html>.

Grant, Taryn. 2020. "COVID-19 Increases Long-Term Care Wait-List by 10% in Nova Scotia." *CBC News*, May 29.<cbc.ca/news/canada/nova-scotia/nova-scotia-long-term-care-wait-list-1.5591054>.

Guye, Alexandrea. 2021. "Long-Term Care Staff in Nova Scotia Still Overworked and Underpaid, MLAS Told." *The Signal*, January 15. <signalhfx.ca/

long-term-care-staff-in-nova-scotia-still-overworked-and-underpaid-mlas-told/>.

Halseth, Regine. 2018. *Overcoming Barriers to Culturally Safe and Appropriate Dementia Care Services and Supports for Indigenous Peoples in Canada*. National Collaborating Centre for Aboriginal Health. <nccah-ccnsa.ca/docs/emerging/RPT-Culturally-Safe-Dementia-Care-Halseth-EN.pdf>.

Hodge, Natalie. 2020. "Tips that Can Help Caregivers Manage Criticism." Home Care Assistance, October 29. <homecareassistancevancouver.ca/handling-caregiver-criticism/>.

Jokogbola, O.R., C. Solomon, and S.L. Wilson. 2018. "Family as Caregiver: Understanding Dementia and Family Relationship." *Advances in Clinical and Translational Research*, 2, 2: 1–5. <laviwilsondsw.com/wp-content/uploads/2017/06/Jokogbola.pdf>.

Justice Laws Website. n.d. "National Strategy for Alzheimer's Disease and Other Dementias Act." Government of Canada. <laws-lois.justice.gc.ca/eng/annualstatutes/2017_19/page-1.html>.

Keefe, J., C. Smith, and G. Archibald. 2018. "Minister's Expert Advisory Panel on Long Term Care." Province of Nova Scotia. <novascotia.ca/dhw/publications/Minister-Expert-Advisory-Panel-on-Long-Term-Care.pdf>.

Leggett, A., B. Bugajski, L. Gitlin, and H. Kales. 2021. "Characterizing Dementia Caregiver Style in Managing Care Challenges: Cognitive and Behavioral Components." *Dementia*, January 31. <journals.sagepub.com/doi/pdf/10.1177/1471301220988233>.

Living Words. n.d. "About the Charity." <livingwords.org.uk/the-charity/>.

Long, C., S. Favaro, and H. Mulder. 2017. "Ambiguous Loss in Dementia Caregiving." Arizona Center on Aging. <uofazcenteronaging.com/care-sheet/providers/ambiguous-loss-dementia-caregiving>.

MacDonald, J.P., V. Ward, and R. Halseth. 2018. *Alzheimer's Disease and Related Dementias in Indigenous Populations in Canada: Prevalence and Risk Factors*. National Collaborating Centre for Aboriginal Health. <nccih.ca/docs/emerging/RPT-Alzheimer-Dementia-MacDonald-Ward-Halseth-EN.pdf>.

Mani, Racheed. 2021. "Depression and Dementia." *Psychology Today*, January 11. <psychologytoday.com/ca/blog/brain-bulletin/202101/depression-and-dementia>.

"Phone-in: The Challenges of Caregiving During the Pandemic." Narrated by Bob Murphy. Maritime Noon. CBC *Radio*, February 4, 2021. <https://www.cbc.ca/listen/live-radio/1-38-maritime-noon>.

McCleary, L., and J. Blain. 2013. "Cultural Values and Family Caregiving for Persons with Dementia." *Indian Journal of Gerontology*, 27, 1: 178–185. <researchgate.net/publication/255754376_Cultural_values_and_family_caregiving_for_persons_with_dementia/link/02e7e520a44d761cb8000000/download>.

Mielke, Michelle M. 2018. "Sex and Gender Differences in Alzheimer Disease Dementia." *Psychiatric Times*, 35, 11. <psychiatrictimes.com/view/sex-and-gender-differences-alzheimer-disease-dementia>.

Molnar, Frank, and C.C. Frank. 2018. "Support of Caregivers of Persons with

Dementia." *Canadian Family Physician*, 64: 294. <cfp.ca/content/cfp/64/4/294.
full.pdf>.

Myette, Mike. 2021. "211 Navigators Refer N.S. Seniors to the Resources They Need."
Saltwire, January 22. <saltwire.com/nova-scotia/more/custom-content/211-
navigators-refer-ns-seniors-to-the-resources-they-need-543938/>.

Nova Scotia Department of Health and Wellness. 2015. *Towards Understanding: A
Dementia Strategy for Nova Scotia*. <novascotia.ca/dhw/dementia/Dementia-
Report-2015.pdf>.

___. 2021. "Nursing Homes and Residential Care Facilities Directory." Government
of Nova Scotia. <novascotia.ca/dhw/ccs/documents/Nursing-Homes-and-
Residential-Care-Directories.pdf>.

Nova Scotia Health Authority. n.d.a. "Geriatric Navigator, Community — DGH."
<cdha.nshealth.ca/geriatric-medicine/geriatric-navigator-community-dgh>.

___. n.d.b. "Centre for Health Care of the Elderly." <cdha.nshealth.ca/
geriatric-medicine/centre-health-care-elderly>.

O'Shaughnessy, M., K. Lee, and T. Lintern. 2010. "Changes in the Couple Relationship
in Dementia Care: Spouse Carers' Experiences." *Dementia*, 9, 2: 237–258 <journals.
sagepub.com/doi/pdf/10.1177/1471301209354021>.

Oliveto, Joe. 2021. "15 Famous Songs about Dementia or Alzheimer's." Cake, March
3. <joincake.com/blog/songs-about-dementia/>.

OM Interactive. n.d. "Mobii Interactive Magic Table For Dementia." <omi.uk/care/
mobii-interactive-table-floor/>.

Ontario Shores Centre for Mental Health Sciences. n.d. "For Caregivers of
People with Dementia." <https://www.ontarioshores.ca/patients___families/
family_and_caregiver_resources/for_caregivers_of_people_with_dementia>.

Pellerin, Brigitte. 2021. "Improving Long-Term Care in Canada." *CBA/ABC National*,
January 18. <nationalmagazine.ca/en-ca/articles/cba-influence/resolutions/2021/
improving-long-term-care-in-canada>.

Pimlott, N.J.G., M. Persaud, N. Drummond, C.A. Cohen, et al. 2009. "Family Physicians
and Dementia in Canada Part 2. Understanding the Challenges of Dementia Care."
Canadian Family Physician, 55, 5: 508–509. <cfp.ca/content/55/5/508.full>.

Province of Nova Scotia. n.d.a. "Continuing Care." <novascotia.ca/dhw/ccs/respite-
care.asp>.

___. n.d.b. "Caregiver Benefit." <novascotia.ca/dhw/ccs/caregiver-benefit.asp>.

___. n.d.c. "Supportive Care." <novascotia.ca/dhw/ccs/FactSheets/Supportive-Care.pdf>.

Quigley, Elizabeth. 2019. "What Does a Dementia-Friendly Town Look Like?" *BBC
News*. October 31. <bbc.com/news/uk-scotland-glasgow-west-50220456>.

RBC Wealth Management. n.d. "Recognizing the Early Signs of Dementia." Eldercare.
<rbcwealthmanagement.com/ca/en/research-insights/recognizing-the-early-
signs-of-dementia/detail/>.

Rosalynn Carter Institute for Caregivers. 2020. "Recalibrating for Caregivers:
Recognizing the Public Health Challenge." <rosalynncarter.org/wp-content/
uploads/2020/10/RCI_Recalibrating-for-Caregivers_2020.pdf>.

Sheets, D., A. Smith, S. MacDonald, E. Phare-Bergh, and R. Bergh. 2020. "In Our
Choir, People with Dementia Sing with Others. Now It's Zooming." May 7.

<thetyee.ca/Culture/2020/05/07/Choir-Dementia-Zooming/>.

Swinkels, J., T. van Tillburg, E., Verbakel, and M. Broese van Groenou. 2019. "Explaining the Gender Gap in the Caregiving Burden of Partner Caregivers." *The Journals of Gerontology: Series B*, 74, 2: 309–317. <academic.oup.com/psychsocgerontology/article/74/2/309/3097902>.

Teahan, Á., A. Lafferty, E. McAuliffe, A. Phelan, et al. 2018. "Resilience in Family Caregiving for People with Dementia: A Systematic Review." *International Journal of Psychiatry*, 33, 12: 1582–1595.

Vanier Institute of the Family. 2020. "In Focus 2020: Caregiving to Older Canadians." February 4. <https://vanierinstitute.ca/in-focus-2020-caregiving-to-older-canadians/>.

The Village. n.d. "Living Here." <thevillagelangley.com>.

West Coast Mommy. n.d. "12 Children's Books to Help Your Child Understand Dementia and Alzheimer's." <thiswestcoastmommy.com/childrens-books-understand-dementia/>.

True North Clinical Research. n.d. "True North Memory Clinics." <truenorthcr.com/memoryclinic/>.

Warchol, Kim. n.d. "Major Neurocognitive Disorder: The DSM-5's New Term for Dementia." Crisis Prevention Institute. <crisisprevention.com/en-CA/Blog/Major-Neurocognitive-Disorder-Dementia>.

Willick, Frances. 2021. "Province to Add 236 Long-Term Care Beds, Replace Hundreds More." *CBC News*, January 29. <cbc.ca/news/canada/nova-scotia/long-term-care-home-renovation-repair-1.5893317>.

Wong, Suzy L., H. Gilmour, and P.L. Ramage-Morin. 2016. "Health Reports: Alzheimer's disease and other dementias in Canada." Statistics Canada. <https://www150.statcan.gc.ca/n1/pub/82-003-x/2016005/article/14613-eng.htm>.

World Health. 2019. "Herbal Chinese Remedies May Help Treat Alzheimer's Disease." July 11. <https://worldhealth.net/news/herbal-chinese-remedies-may-help-treat-alzheimers-disease/>.

World Health Organization. 2017. *Global Action Plan on the Public Health Response to Dementia 2017–2025*. <who.int/mental_health/neurology/dementia/action_plan_2017_2025/en/>.

Youell, J., J.E.M. Callaghan, and K. Buchanan. 2015. "'I Don't Know if You Want to Know This': Carers' Understandings of Intimacy in Long-Term Relationships when One Partner Has Dementia." *Ageing and Society*, 36, 5: 1–22.

Zaugg, Julie. 2019. "China Approves Seaweed-based Alzheimer's Drug. It's the First New One in 17 Years." *CNN*, November 5. <https://www.cnn.com/2019/11/03/health/china-alzheimers-drug-intl-hnk-scli>.

Zimmer, Eric. 2019. "A Look Inside: Canada's First 'Dementia Village.'" *The Daily Hive*, July 23. <dailyhive.com/vancouver/canada-first-dementia-village-langley-bc-photos-july-2019>.

Zhou, Y., A. O'Hara, E. Ishado, S. Borson, and T. Sadak. 2019. "Behavioral Markers of Resilience in Care Partners of Persons with Dementia: A Thematic Analysis from a Scoping Review." *Innovation in Aging*, 3, 1: S595.